Renal Diet Cookbook for Beginners and the Newly Diagnosed

Low Sodium, Low Potassium & Low Phosphorus Renal Diet Recipes to Manage Your Kidney Disease and Avoid Dialysis.

Viktoria McCartney

Introduction

A renal diet is a diet, especially for patients who are suffering from kidney health problems. What you eat plays a vital role in keeping your kidneys healthy and functioning. This diet helps your kidneys to rest and balances the pH levels of the blood. A delicious approach to the prevention and management of kidney problems with handpicked renal diet recipes. The first step to slow down the progression of kidney disease is to limit your sodium, potassium, phosphate and protein intake. This guide has been prepared to help renal patients prepare all meals without much hassle.

One of the challenges faced by most kidney patients is finding simple, delicious Chronic Kidney Disease (CKD) recipes to help them manage the levels of chemicals and fluid in their blood. This renal diet cookbook helps to find a stable ground between savoring the taste of your food and making the required dietary adjustment. The recipes in this cookbook have low sodium, low potassium, low phosphorus and a controlled amount of healthy protein. This book will help you to improve your knowledge of the kidney diet, and you will have many easy and tasty alternative recipes.

Chapter 1 Chronic Kidney Disease

Kidneys are important organs for the human body. They filter out excess water, waste products, and other impurities of the blood. Chronic kidney disease or CKD means your kidneys are damaged and can't filter blood properly. The kidney damage can cause waste to build up in your body. CKD causes many health problem.

Who is at risk of developing CKD?

1. Diabetes: People with diabetes are prone to CKD. Data shows that about one-third of diabetic patients have CKD.
2. High blood pressure: About 1 in 5 adults with high blood pressure has CKD.
3. Heart disease: Recent research shows that there is a link between high blood pressure and kidney disease. People with kidney disease are at a higher risk of heart disease and people with heart disease are at a higher risk of kidney disease.
4. Family history of kidney failure: People with a family history are at risk for CKD.

Besides this there are other risk factors including

- Being Asian-American, Native American, and African-American
- Smoking
- Old age
- Obesity

Symptoms of CKD

Early stages of chronic kidney disease may not have any symptoms. It is because even if your kidney is damaged, it can still do enough work to keep you healthy. The blood and urine tests are the only ways to know if you have kidney disease.

Symptoms of advanced CKD

- Weight loss
- Vomiting
- Trouble concentrating
- Sleep problems
- Shortness of breath
- Nausea
- Muscle cramps
- Loss of appetite
- Increased or decreased urination
- Headaches
- Feeling tired
- Itching or numbness
- Dry skin
- Chest pain

A brief snapshot of each stage:

Stage 1: Considered the normal or high risk of developing CKD. The Glomerular Filtration Rate (GFR) falls > 90 mL/min.

Stage 2: Considered as mild CKD. The GFR falls in the range of 60-89 mL/min.

Stage 3: Moderate CKD which ranges from 45-59 mL/min.

Stage 4: Severe Chronic Kidney disease. Rates fall between 15-29 mL/min.

Stage 5: Final/end-stage of the renal disease which calls for surgery or dialysis. Also called End Stage Renal Disease (ESRD). The GFR levels, in this case, fall below 15 mL/min.

Chapter 2 The Renal Diet

Depending on the stage of your kidney disease, blood-work results, type of treatment and whether you have high blood pressure or diabetes, your renal diet "prescription" will vary. In this chapter, we are going to discuss important macronutrients, vitamins, and minerals, including:

- Potassium
- Phosphorus
- Calories
- Protein
- Fats
- Sodium
- Carbohydrates
- Vitamins/Minerals
- Fluids

Potassium

Potassium is a crucial mineral that is required for the body to keep your heart strong and healthy. Healthy kidneys remove excess potassium through urination. However, when your kidneys are not working properly, they can't remove the potassium, so it builds up in the blood. Having too much or too little potassium in the blood can be dangerous to the body. Your potassium needs may vary depending on how well your kidneys are functioning. If you are receiving dialysis, you need to keep your potassium intake between 2,000 and 3,000 milligrams per day.

Phosphorus

Healthy kidneys can remove extra phosphorus from the blood. However, when the kidneys are failing, phosphorus builds up into the blood and may cause problems. If you have chronic kidney disease or are receiving dialysis, phosphorous in the diet should be limited to between 800 and 1,000 milligrams per day.

Calories

Your body needs more calories when you develop kidney disease, especially if you are on dialysis. In both chronic kidney disease and with dialysis, daily calorie requirements are 30 to 35 calories per kilogram of body weight. So, if your weight is 150 pounds, you need to consume 2,000 calories each day.

Protein

If you are in stage 1,2, or 3 of chronic kidney disease, your protein intake will be limited to 12 to 15% of your calorie intake each day. If you are in stage 4 of chronic kidney disease, your protein intake will be reduced to 10% of your daily calorie intake. People who are on dialysis should eat about 1.2 grams of protein per kilogram of body weight each day. So, if you are 150 pounds, consume 82 grams of protein per day.

Fats

If your doctor recommends you to eat 2,000 calories, your calories from fat should be limited to 600 calories, it is about 70 grams of fat. You need to consume healthy fats such as olive oil, and fatty fish such as tuna and salmon.

Sodium

When your kidneys do not work well, sodium starts to build up and can cause thirst, fluid-weight gain, and high blood pressure. You need to make some dietary modifications if you are in the early stages of chronic kidney disease. If you have stage 5 chronic kidney disease and require dialysis, then follow a low-sodium diet and do not consume more than 1,500 milligrams of sodium.

Carbohydrates and fiber

Some carb-rich foods also contain fiber and this plays an important role in improving your kidney disease condition. Fiber can help reduce kidney disease symptoms.

Whole Grains

Whole grains in moderation can be very helpful for kidney disease patients.

Vitamin and Mineral Supplements

If you have kidney disease, then over-the-counter multivitamins are not good for your health. You need to avoid or limit vitamins A, E, and K because levels of these vitamins build up in the body as kidney function decreases. Talk with your physician about vitamin and mineral supplements.

Fluids

Depending on your stage of kidney disease, you may need to limit the fluids you drink.

How to avoid "double trouble" foods

Double trouble foods – those that are high in both potassium and phosphorus including milk, and dairy foods, chocolate, nuts and seeds. These foods are best to avoid or use in small amounts.

Chapter 3 Preparing for The Diet

Reading food labels is essential to making healthy food choices for your kidneys. The nutrition facts label will serve as a guide to help you make healthier choices.

Here are some words to look for when reading the nutrition facts label:

- Claims such as "low in saturated fat" or "fat-free".
- "no-salt-added", "sodium-free", "sodium-restricted", and "unsalted".

Check the ingredient list for phosphorus or for the words that start with "phos". Check the ingredient list for potassium.

Nutrition Facts

4 servings per container
Serving size 1 1/2 cup (208g)

Amount per serving **Calories**	**240**
	% Daily Value*
Total Fat 4g	**5%**
Saturated Fat 1.5g	**8%**
Trans Fat 0g	
Cholesterol 5mg	**2%**
Sodium 430mg	**19%**
Total Carbohydrate 46g	**17%**
Dietary Fiber 7g	**25%**
Total Sugars 4g	
Includes 2g Added Sugars	**4%**
Protein 11g	
Vitamin D 2mcg	10%
Calcium 260mg	20%
Iron 6mg	35%
Potassium 240mg	6%

* The % Daily Value (DV) tells you how much a nutrient in a serving of food contributes to a daily diet. 2,000 calories a day is used for general nutrition advice.

Stocking a kidney-friendly pantry

The following is a list as a guide for your kitchen staples, Grocery list or a kidney-friendly pantry

Meat and meat substitutes

Beef	Chicken	Eggs	Egg substitute
Fish	Lamb	Pork, chops/ roast	Tofu
Tuna, canned	Turkey	Veal	

Vegetables

Alfalfa sprouts	Arugula	Asparagus	Bean sprouts
Beets, canned	Cabbage, green/red	Carrots	Cauliflower
Celery	Chiles	Chives	Coleslaw
Corn	Cucumber	Eggplant	Endive
Ginger root	Green beans	Lettuce	Onions
Parsley	Radishes	Spaghetti squash	Turnips

Vegetables, mixed	Water chestnuts, canned		

Fruits

Apple juice	Apples	Applesauce	Apricot nectar
Apricots, canned	Blackberries	Cherries	Cranberries
Cranberry juice	Cranberry sauce	Figs, fresh	Fruit cocktail
Grapefruit	Grapefruit juice	Grapes	Lemon
Lime	Peaches	Peach nectar	
Pears, canned	Pineapple	Raspberries	Strawberries
Tangerines	Watermelon	Plums	

Bread and Cereals

Bagels, plain/blueberry	Bread, white/French/Italian	Cereals, Kellogg's Corn Flakes	Cereals, Cheerios
Cereals, Corn Chex	Couscous	Crackers, unsalted	Dinner rolls
English muffins	Grits	Hamburger/hot dog rolls	Pasta
Melba toast	Noodles	Oyster crackers	Pita bread
Pretzels, unsalted	Rice, brown/white	Spaghetti	Tortillas

Fats

Butter	Canola oil	Cream cheese	Margarine
Mayonnaise	Miracle Whip	Nondairy creamers	Olive oil

Sweets

Animal crackers	Angel food cake	Candy corn	Chewing gum
Cotton candy	Crispy rice treats	Graham crackers	Gumdrops
Gummy bears	Hard candy	Hot Tamales candy	Jell-O
Jelly beans	Jolly Rancher	Lemon cake	Life Savers
Marshmallows	Newtons (fig, strawberry, apple, blueberry)	Pie (apple, berry, cherry, lemon, peach)	Pound cake
Rice cakes	Vanilla wafers		

Beverages

7UP	Coffee	Cream soda	Fruit punch
Ginger ale	Grape soda	Hi-C	Lemon-lime soda
Lemonade	Orange soda	Root beer	Tea

Dairy and Dairy Alternatives

Almond milk	Coffee-mate	Mocha Mix
Rice Dream	Rich's Coffee Rich	

Other

Apple butter	Corn syrup	Honey	Jam
Jelly	Maple syrup	Sugar, brown or white	Sugar, powdered

Chapter 4 Tips

Tips on controlling your phosphorous

Here is what you should do to maintain a balanced level of phosphorous:

- Limit the consumption of foods like poultry, meats, fish and dairy
- Limit the intake of certain dairy products like yogurt and cheese; you should not exceed 4 oz. per serving
- Avoid black beans, lima beans, red beans, garbanzo beans, white beans and black-eyed peas.
- Avoid unrefined, whole and dark grains.
- Stay away from refrigerator dough
- Avoid dried fruits and vegetables
- Avoid chocolate
- Avoid sodas that are dark-colored
- Make sure to take your phosphate binders with your snacks and meals.
- The renal diet limits the intake of phosphorus to 1000mg per day

Tips on controlling your protein

Make sure to consume high-quality proteins. Eat about 7 to 8 oz. of protein per day. Pork, beef, turkey, veal; chicken and eggs have high amounts of protein.

Tips on controlling your fluid intake

- Use 1 cup or glass in order to divide your fluid intake per day. You can also write a record of your fluid intake.

- Always avoid any type of salty food and never add extra salt to your meals.
- Avoid processed meats, fast foods and canned foods
- You can add lemon juice to the water you want to drink instead
- You can rinse your mouth with a mouthwash from time to time
- Avoid overheating
- Maintain your blood sugar at a balanced level

Eating Out

Look out for small or half portions and ask your server for your foods to be cooked without extra salt, butter or sauce. Avoid fried foods, instead, embrace poached or grilled food. If you know, you are going out to eat, plan ahead. Look at the restaurant menu beforehand online.

Eating at social gatherings (such as birthdays, weddings, picnics, and barbecues)

1. Don't go hungry: Have a snack before you leave the house.
2. Avoid high-sodium foods: Avoid foods such as hot dogs or sausages. Choose lower-sodium foods such as chicken and hamburgers.
3. Limit alcohol: Speak with your physician first about drinking alcohol.
4. Food safety is important: Keep food at safe temperatures, wash well, and use separate cutting boards for raw and cooked meats.
5. Plan ahead: Plan your menus.

FAQ

Q: What is the maximum potassium daily limit?

A: When following a renal diet, you ideally want to make sure that potassium levels are below 250mg/per serving or up to 7% of the food's total nutritional value.

Q: Can I lose weight with a renal diet?

A: The amount of calories that you need to take depends on your age, gender, health status, and weight goal. If you want to lose weight on your renal diet plan, then discuss it with a nutritionist.

Q: Does my CKD stage count when following a renal diet?

A: Yes. In earlier stages (1 to 3), it is fine to consume low to moderate amounts of sodium, potassium, and phosphorus, while your fluid intake should be up to 2.5 liters per day. However, if you are in dialysis, then you have to limit all the above minerals.

Q: Is it okay to take caffeine in a renal diet?

A: During the first three stages of CKD, a caffeine-based drink is perfectly fine. You may drink up to 2 cups of coffee per day without any worries.

Q: How about over the counter medication?

A: Counter medication/painkillers like aspirin and ibuprofen are not indicated for CKD patients. Any drug that belongs in the nonsteroidal anti-inflammatory drugs category should be avoided.

Chapter 5 Breakfast Recipes

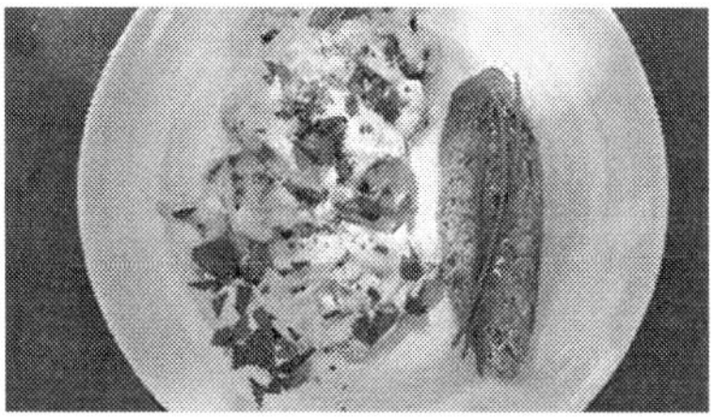

Cheesy Scrambled Eggs with Fresh Herbs

Prep time: 15 minutes	Cook time: 10 minutes	Servings: 4

Ingredients

- Eggs – 3
- Egg whites – 2
- Cream cheese – ½ cup
- Unsweetened rice milk – ¼ cup
- Chopped scallion – 1 Tbsp. green part only
- Chopped fresh tarragon – 1 Tbsp.
- Unsalted butter – 2 Tbsps.
- Ground black pepper to taste

Method

1. In a bowl, whisk the eggs, egg whites, cream cheese, rice milk, scallions, and tarragon until mixed and smooth.
2. Melt the butter in a skillet.
3. Pour in the egg mixture and cook, stirring, for 5 minutes or until the eggs are thick and curds creamy.

4. Season with pepper and serve.

Nutritional Facts Per Serving

- Calories: 221
- Fat: 19g
- Carb: 3g
- Phosphorus: 119mg
- Potassium: 140mg
- Sodium: 193mg
- Protein: 8g

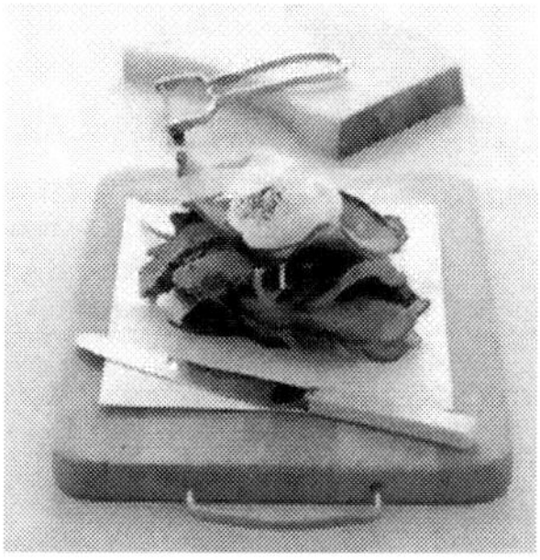

Turkey and Spinach Scramble on Melba Toast

Prep time: 2 minutes	Cook time: 15 minutes	Servings: 2

Ingredients

- Extra virgin olive oil – 1 tsp
- Raw spinach – 1 cup
- Garlic – ½ clove, minced
- Nutmeg – 1 tsp. grated

- Cooked and diced turkey breast – 1 cup
- Melba toast – 4 slices
- Balsamic vinegar – 1 tsp.

Method

1. Heat a skillet over medium heat and add oil.
2. Add turkey and heat through for 6 to 8 minutes.
3. Add spinach, garlic, and nutmeg and stir-fry for 6 minutes more.
4. Plate up the Melba toast and top with spinach and turkey scramble.
5. Drizzle with balsamic vinegar and serve.

Nutritional Facts Per Serving

- Calories: 301
- Fat: 19g
- Carb: 12g
- Phosphorus: 215mg
- Potassium: 269mg
- Sodium: 360mg
- Protein: 19g

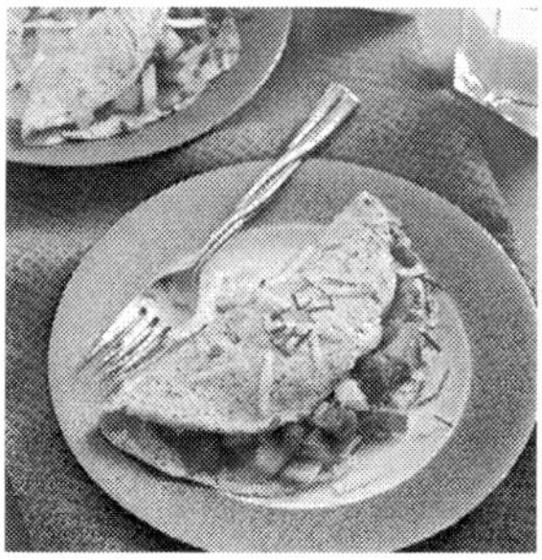

Vegetable Omelet

Prep time: 15 minutes	Cook time: 10 minutes	Servings: 3

Ingredients

- Egg whites – 4
- Egg – 1
- Chopped fresh parsley – 2 Tbsps.
- Water – 2 Tbsps.
- Olive oil spray
- Chopped and boiled red bell pepper – ½ cup
- Chopped scallion – ¼ cup, both green and white parts
- Ground black pepper

Method

1. Whisk together the egg, egg whites, parsley, and water until well blended. Set aside.
2. Spray a skillet with olive oil spray and place over medium heat.
3. Sauté the peppers and scallion for 3 minutes or until softened.

4. Pour the egg mixture into the skillet over vegetables and cook, swirling the skillet, for 2 minutes or until the edges start to set. Cook until set.
5. Season with black pepper and serve.

Nutritional Facts Per Serving

- Calories: 77
- Fat: 3g
- Carb: 2g
- Phosphorus: 67mg
- Potassium: 194mg
- Sodium: 229mg
- Protein: 12g

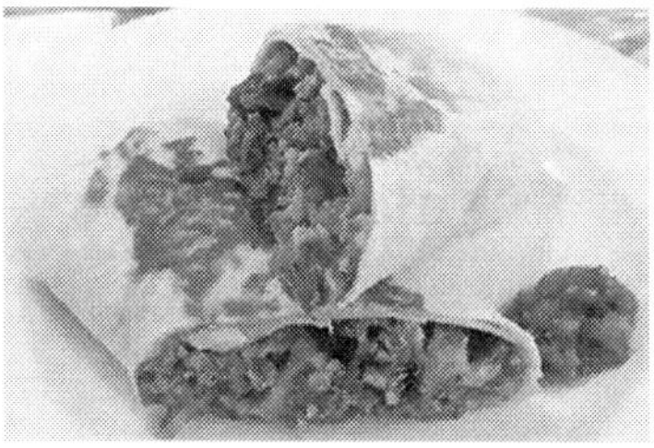

Mexican Style Burritos

Prep time: 5 minutes	Cook time: 15 minutes	Servings: 2

Ingredients

- Olive oil – 1 Tbsp.
- Corn tortillas – 2
- Red onion – ¼ cup, chopped

- Red bell peppers – ¼ cup, chopped
- Red chili – ½, deseeded and chopped
- Eggs – 2
- Juice of 1 lime
- Cilantro – 1 Tbsp. chopped

Method

1. Turn the broiler to medium heat and place the tortillas underneath for 1 to 2 minutes on each side or until lightly toasted.
2. Remove and keep the broiler on.
3. Heat the oil in a skillet and sauté onion, chili and bell peppers for 5 to 6 minutes or until soft.
4. Crack the eggs over the top of the onions and peppers and place skillet under the broiler for 5 to 6 minutes or until the eggs are cooked.
5. Serve half the eggs and vegetables on top of each tortilla and sprinkle with cilantro and lime juice to serve.

Nutritional Facts Per Serving

- Calories: 202
- Fat: 13g
- Carb: 19g
- Phosphorus: 184mg
- Potassium: 233mg
- Sodium: 77mg

- Protein: 9g

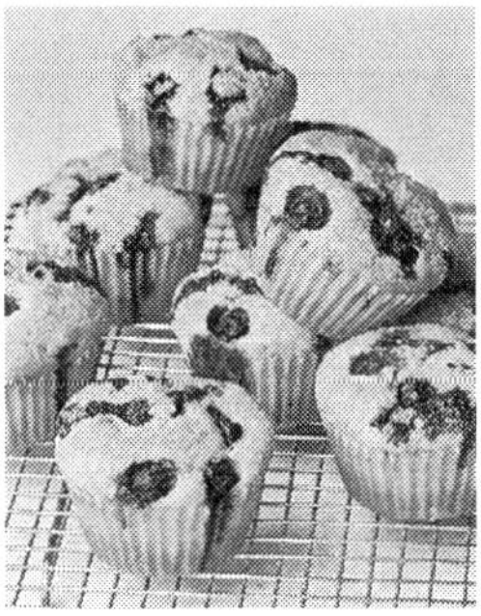

Blueberry Muffins

Prep time: 15 minutes	Cook time: 30 minutes	Servings: 12

Ingredients

- Unsweetened rice milk – 2 cups
- Apple cider vinegar – 1 Tbsp.
- All-purpose flour – 3 ½ cups
- Granulated sugar – 1 cup
- Baking soda substitute – 1 Tbsp.
- Ground cinnamon – 1 tsp.
- Ground nutmeg – ½ tsp.
- Pinch ground ginger
- Canola oil – ½ cup
- Pure vanilla extract – 2 Tbsps.
- Fresh blueberries – 2 ½ cups

Method

1. Preheat the oven to 375F.
2. Line the cups of a muffin pan with paper liners. Set aside.
3. In a small bowl, stir together the rice milk and vinegar. Set aside for 10 minutes.
4. In a large bowl, stir together the sugar, flour, baking soda, cinnamon, nutmeg, and ginger until well mixed.
5. Add the oil and vanilla to the milk mixture and stir to blend.
6. Add the milk mixture to the dry ingredients and stir until just combined.
7. Fold in the blueberries. Spoon the muffin batter evenly into the cups.
8. Bake the muffins for 25 to 30 minutes or until golden and a toothpick inserted comes out clean.
9. Cool for 15 minutes and serve.

Nutritional Facts Per Serving

- Calories: 331
- Fat: 11g
- Carb: 52g
- Phosphorus: 90mg
- Potassium: 89mg
- Sodium: 35mg
- Protein: 6g

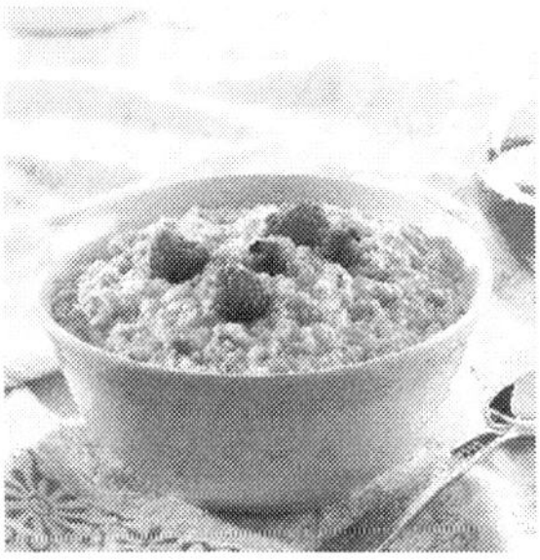

Bulgur, Couscous and Buckwheat Cereal

Prep time: 10 minutes	Cook time: 25 minutes	Servings: 4

Ingredients

- Water – 2 ¼ cups
- Vanilla rice milk – 1 ¼ cups
- Uncooked bulgur – 6 Tbsps.
- Uncooked whole buckwheat – 2 Tbsps.
- Sliced apple – 1 cup
- Plain uncooked couscous – 6 Tbsps.
- Ground cinnamon – ½ tsp.

Method

1. In a saucepan, heat the water and milk over medium heat.
2. Bring to a boil, and add the bulgur, buckwheat, and apple.
3. Reduce the heat to low and simmer, occasionally stirring until the bulgur is tender, about 20 to 25 minutes.
4. Remove the saucepan from the heat and stir in the couscous and cinnamon.

5. Let the saucepan stand, covered, for 10 minutes.
6. Fluff the cereal with a fork before serving.

Nutritional Facts Per Serving

- Calories: 159
- Fat: 1g
- Carb: 34g
- Phosphorus: 130mg
- Potassium: 116mg
- Sodium: 33mg
- Protein: 4g

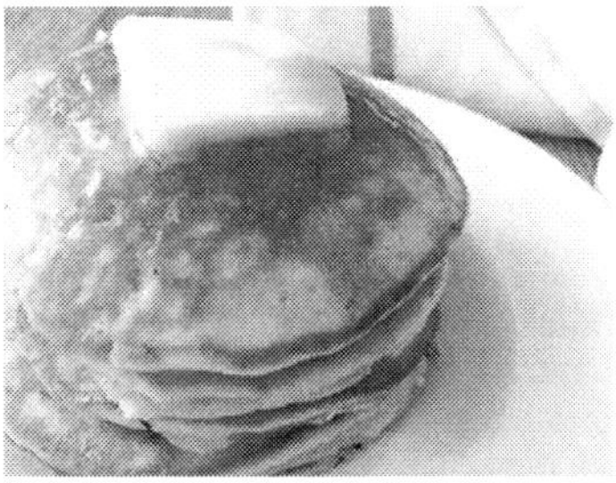

Sweet Pancakes

Prep time: 10 minutes	Cook time: 5 minutes	Servings: 5

Ingredients

- All-purpose flour – 1 cup
- Granulated sugar – 1 Tbsp.
- Baking powder – 2 tsps.
- Egg whites – 2

- Almond milk - 1 cup
- Olive oil - 2 Tbsps.
- Maple extract – 1 Tbsp.

Method

1. Mix the flour, sugar and baking powder in a bowl.
2. Make a well in the center and place to one side.
3. In another bowl, mix the egg whites, milk, oil, and maple extract.
4. Add the egg mixture to the well and gently mix until a batter is formed.
5. Heat skillet over medium heat.
6. Add 1/5 of the batter to the pan and cook 2 minutes on each side or until the pancake is golden.
7. Repeat with the remaining batter and serve.

Nutritional Facts Per Serving

- Calories: 178
- Fat: 6g
- Carb: 25g
- Phosphorus: 116mg
- Potassium: 126mg
- Sodium: 297mg
- Protein: 6g

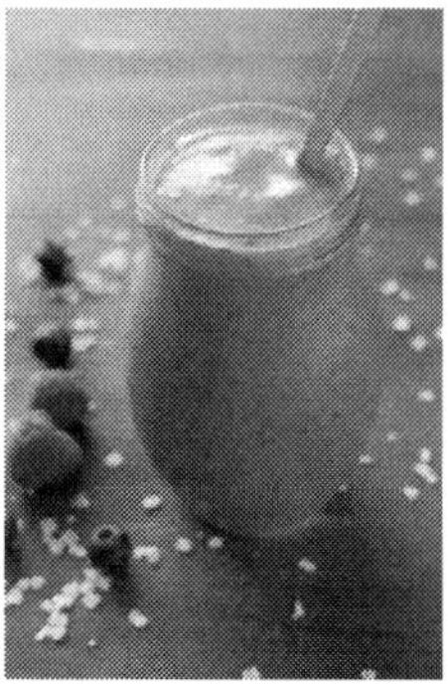

Breakfast Smoothie

Prep time: 15 minutes	Cook time: 0 minutes	Servings: 2

Ingredients

- Frozen blueberries – 1 cup
- Pineapple chunks – ½ cup
- English cucumber – ½ cup
- Apple – ½
- Water – ½ cup

Method

1. Put the pineapple, blueberries, cucumber, apple, and water in a blender and blend until thick and smooth.
2. Pour into 2 glasses and serve.

Nutritional Facts Per Serving

- Calories: 87
- Fat: g
- Carb: 22g

- Phosphorus: 28mg
- Potassium: 192mg
- Sodium: 3mg
- Protein: 0.7g

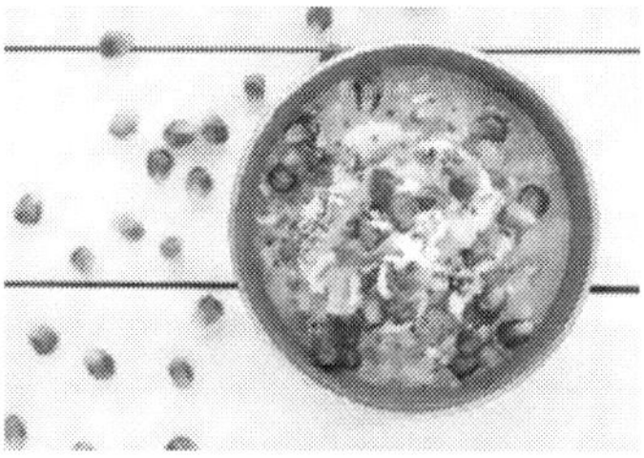

Buckwheat and Grapefruit Porridge

Prep time: 5 minutes	Cook time: 20 minutes	Servings: 2

Ingredients

- Buckwheat – ½ cup
- Grapefruit – ¼, chopped
- Honey – 1 Tbsp.
- Almond milk – 1 ½ cups
- Water – 2 cups

Method

1. Bring the water to a boil on the stove. Add the buckwheat and place the lid on the pan.
2. Lower heat slightly and simmer for 7 to 10 minutes, checking to ensure water does not dry out.
3. When most of the water is absorbed, remove and set aside for 5 minutes.

4. Drain any excess water from the pan and stir in almond milk, heating through for 5 minutes.
5. Add the honey and grapefruit.
6. Serve.

Nutritional Facts Per Serving

- Calories: 231
- Fat: 4g
- Carb: 43g
- Phosphorus: 165mg
- Potassium: 370mg
- Sodium: 135mg

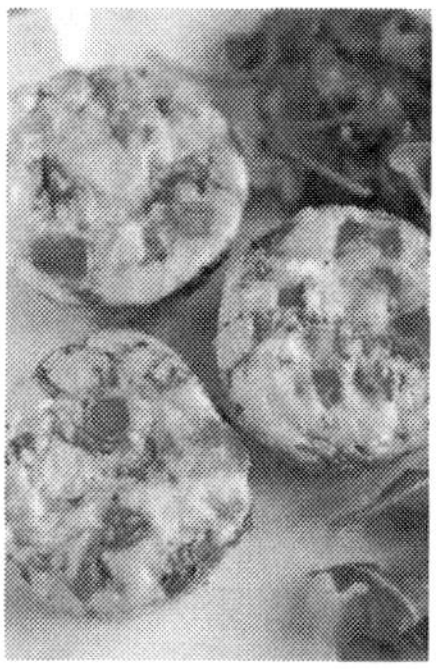

Egg and Veggie Muffins

Prep time: 15 minutes	Cook time: 20 minutes	Servings: 4

Ingredients

- Cooking spray
- Eggs – 4
- Unsweetened rice milk – 2 Tbsp.

- Sweet onion – ½, chopped
- Red bell pepper – ½, chopped
- Pinch red pepper flakes
- Pinch ground black pepper

Method

1. Preheat the oven to 350F.
2. Spray 4 muffin pans with cooking spray. Set aside.
3. In a bowl, whisk together the milk, eggs, onion, red pepper, parsley, red pepper flakes, and black pepper until mixed.
4. Pour the egg mixture into prepared muffin pans.
5. Bake until the muffins are puffed and golden, about 18 to 20 minutes.
6. serve

Nutritional Facts Per Serving

- Calories: 84
- Fat: 5g
- Carb: 3g
- Phosphorus: 110mg
- Potassium: 117mg
- Sodium: 75mg
- Protein: 7g

Chapter 6 Lunch Recipes

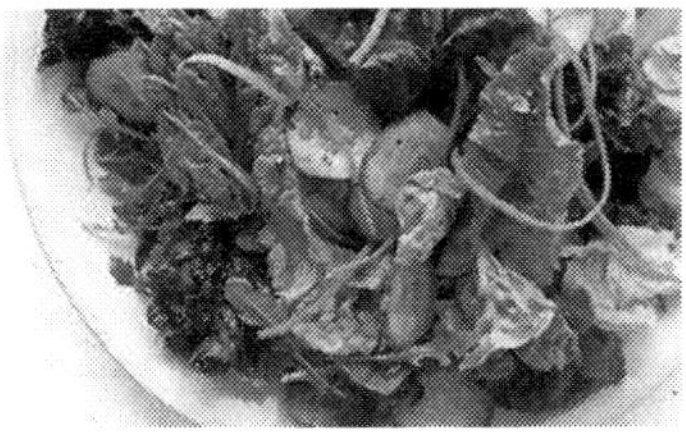

Salad with Vinaigrette

Prep time: 25 minutes	Cook time: 0 minutes	Servings: 4

Ingredients for the vinaigrette

- Olive oil – ½ cup
- Balsamic vinegar - 4 Tbsps.
- Chopped fresh oregano – 2 Tbsps.
- Pinch red pepper flakes
- Ground black pepper

For the salad

- Shredded green leaf lettuce – 4 cups
- Carrot – 1, shredded
- Fresh green beans – ¾ cup, cut into 1-inch pieces
- Large radishes – 3, sliced thin

Method

1. To make the vinaigrette: put the vinaigrette ingredients in a bowl and whisk.
2. To make the salad, in a bowl, toss together the carrot, lettuce, green beans, and radishes.

3. Add the vinaigrette to the vegetables and toss to coat.
4. Arrange the salad on plates and serve.

Nutritional Facts Per Serving

- Calories: 273
- Fat: 27g
- Carb: 7g
- Phosphorus: 30mg
- Potassium: 197mg
- Sodium: 27mg
- Protein: 1g

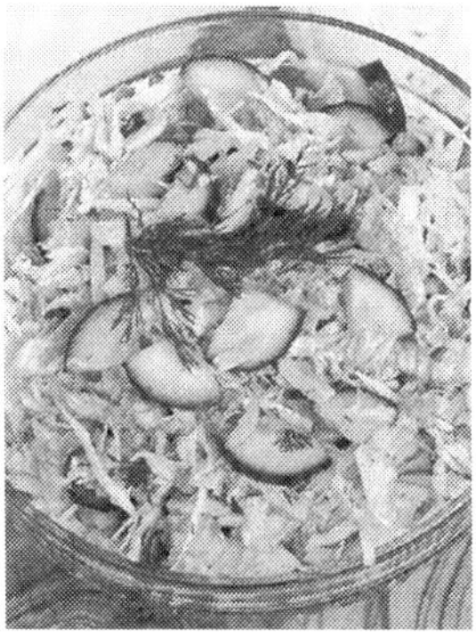

Salad with Lemon Dressing

Prep time: 10 minutes	Cook time: 0 minutes	Servings: 4

Ingredients

- Heavy cream – ¼ cup
- Freshly squeezed lemon juice – ¼ cup

- Granulated sugar – 2 Tbsps.
- Chopped fresh dill – 2 Tbsps.
- Finely chopped scallion – 2 Tbsps. green part only
- Ground black pepper – ¼ tsp.
- English cucumber – 1, sliced thin
- Shredded green cabbage – 2 cups

Method

1. In a small bowl, stir together the lemon juice, cream, sugar, dill, scallion, and pepper until well blended.
2. In a large bowl, toss together the cucumber and cabbage.
3. Place the salad in the refrigerator and chill for 1 hour.
4. Stir before serving.

Nutritional Facts Per Serving

- Calories: 99
- Fat: 6g
- Carb: 13g
- Phosphorus: 38mg
- Potassium: 200mg
- Sodium: 14mg
- Protein: 2g

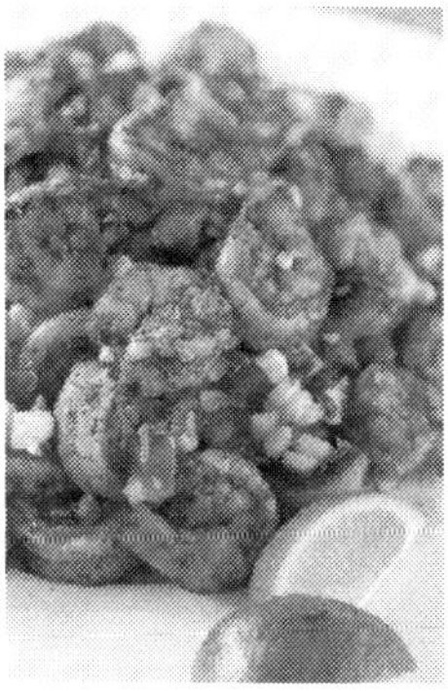

Shrimp with Salsa

Prep time: 15 minutes	Cook time: 10 minutes	Servings: 4

Ingredients

- Olive oil – 2 Tbsp.
- Large shrimp – 6 ounces, peeled and deveined, tails left on
- Minced garlic – 1 tsp.
- Chopped English cucumber – ½ cup
- Chopped mango – ½ cup
- Zest of 1 lime
- Juice of 1 lime
- Ground black pepper
- Lime wedges for garnish

Method

1. Soak 4 wooden skewers in water for 30 minutes.
2. Preheat the barbecue to medium heat.

3. In a bowl, toss together the olive oil, shrimp, and garlic.
4. Thread the shrimp onto the skewers, about 4 shrimp per skewer.
5. In a bowl, stir together the mango, cucumber, lime zest, and lime juice, and season the salsa lightly with pepper. Set aside.
6. Grill the shrimp for 10 minutes, turning once or until the shrimp is opaque and cooked through.
7. Season the shrimp lightly with pepper.
8. Serve the shrimp on the cucumber salsa with lime wedges on the side.

Nutritional Facts Per Serving

- Calories: 120
- Fat: 8g
- Carb: 4g
- Phosphorus: 91mg
- Potassium: 129mg
- Sodium: 60mg
- Protein: 9g

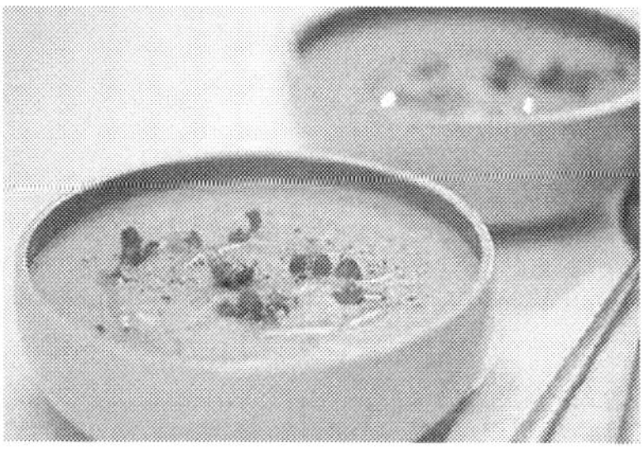

Cauliflower Soup

Prep time: 20 minutes	Cook time: 30	Servings: 6

Ingredients

- Unsalted butter – 1 tsp.
- Sweet onion – 1 small, chopped
- Minced garlic – 2 tsps.
- Small head cauliflower – 1, cut into small florets
- Curry powder – 2 tsps.
- Water to cover the cauliflower
- Light sour cream – ½ cup
- Chopped fresh cilantro – 3 Tbsps.

Method

1. In a large saucepan, heat the butter over a medium-high heat and sauté the onion-garlic for about 3 minutes or until softened.
2. Add the cauliflower, water, and curry powder.
3. Bring the soup to a boil, then reduce the heat to low and simmer for 20 minutes or until the cauliflower is tender.

4. Puree the soup until creamy and smooth with a hand mixer.
5. Transfer the soup back into a saucepan and stir in the sour cream and cilantro.
6. Heat the soup on medium heat for 5 minutes or until warmed through.

Nutritional Facts Per Serving

- Calories: 33
- Fat: 2g
- Carb: 4g
- Phosphorus: 30mg
- Potassium: 167mg
- Sodium: 22mg
- Protein: 1g

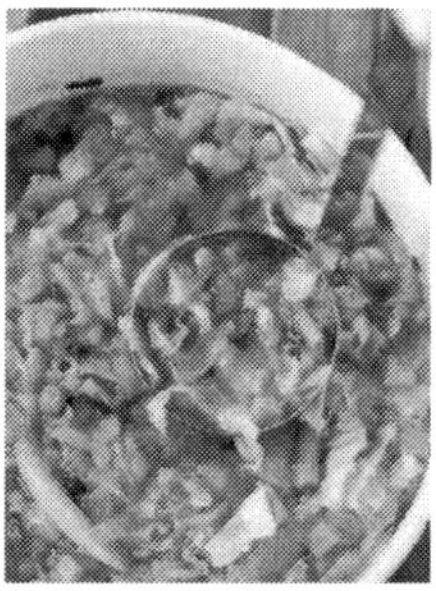

Cabbage Stew

Prep time: 20 minutes	Cook time: 35 minutes	Servings: 6

Ingredients

- Unsalted butter – 1 tsp.

- Large sweet onion - ½, chopped
- Minced garlic – 1 tsp.
- Shredded green cabbage – 6 cups
- Celery stalks - 3, chopped with leafy tops
- Scallion – 1, both green and white parts, chopped
- Chopped fresh parsley – 2 Tbsps.
- Freshly squeezed lemon juice – 2 Tbsps.
- Chopped fresh thyme – 1 Tbsp.
- Chopped savory – 1 tsp.
- Chopped fresh oregano – 1 tsp.
- Water
- Fresh green beans – 1 cup, cut into 1-inch pieces
- Ground black pepper

Method

1. Melt the butter in a pot.
2. Sauté the onion and garlic in the melted butter for 3 minutes, or until the vegetables are softened.
3. Add the celery, cabbage, scallion, parsley, lemon juice, thyme, savory, and oregano to the pot, add enough water to cover the vegetables by 4 inches.
4. Bring the soup to a boil. Reduce the heat to low and simmer the soup for 25 minutes or until the vegetables are tender.
5. Add the green beans and simmer for 3 minutes.

6. Season with pepper.

Nutritional Facts Per Serving

- Calories: 33
- Fat: 1g
- Carb: 6g
- Phosphorus: 29mg
- Potassium: 187mg
- Sodium: 20mg
- Protein: 1g

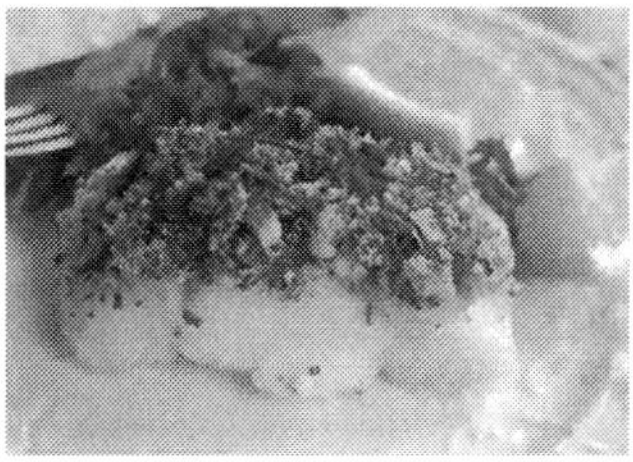

Baked Haddock

Prep time: 10 minutes	Cook time: 20 minutes	Servings: 4

Ingredients

- Bread crumbs – ½ cup
- Chopped fresh parsley – 3 Tbsps.
- Lemon zest – 1 Tbsp.
- Chopped fresh thyme – 1 tsp.
- Ground black pepper – ¼ tsp.

- Melted unsalted butter – 1 Tbsp.
- Haddock fillets – 12-ounces, deboned and skinned

Method

1. Preheat the oven to 350F.
2. In a bowl, stir together the parsley, breadcrumbs, lemon zest, thyme, and pepper until well combined.
3. Add the melted butter and toss until the mixture resembles coarse crumbs.
4. Place the haddock on a baking sheet and spoon the bread crumb mixture on top, pressing down firmly.
5. Bake the haddock in the oven for 20 minutes or until the fish is just cooked through and flakes off in chunks when pressed.

Nutritional Facts Per Serving

- Calories: 143
- Fat: 4g
- Carb: 10g
- Phosphorus: 216mg
- Potassium: 285mg
- Sodium: 281mg
- Protein: 16g

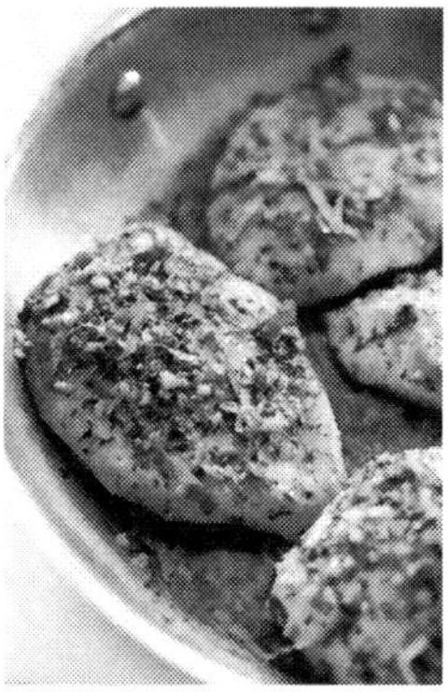

Herbed Chicken

Prep time: 20 minutes	Cook time: 15 minutes	Servings: 4

Ingredients

- Boneless, skinless chicken breast – 12 ounces, cut into 8 strips
- Egg white – 1
- Water – 2 Tbsps. divided
- Breadcrumbs – ½ cup
- Unsalted butter – ¼ cup, divided
- Juice of 1 lemon
- Zest of 1 lemon
- Fresh chopped basil – 1 Tbsp.
- Fresh chopped thyme – 1 tsp.
- Lemon slices, for garnish

Method

1. Place the chicken strips between 2 sheets of plastic wrap and pound each flat with a rolling pin.
2. In a bowl, whisk together the egg and 1 tbsp. water.
3. Put the breadcrumbs in another bowl.
4. Dredge the chicken strips, one at a time, in the egg, then the breadcrumbs and set the breaded strips aside on a plate.
5. In a large skillet over medium heat, melt 2 tbsps. of the butter.
6. Cook the strips in the butter for 3 minutes, turning once, or until they are golden and cooked through. Transfer the chicken to a plate.
7. Add the lemon zest, lemon juice, basil, thyme, and remaining 1 tbsp. water to the skillet and stir until the mixture simmers.
8. Remove the sauce from the heat and stir in the remaining 2 tbsps. butter.
9. Serve the chicken with the lemon sauce drizzled over the top and garnished with lemon slices.

Nutritional Facts Per Serving

- Calories: 255
- Fat: 14g
- Carb: 11g
- Phosphorus: 180mg
- Potassium: 321mg
- Sodium: 261mg
- Protein: 20g

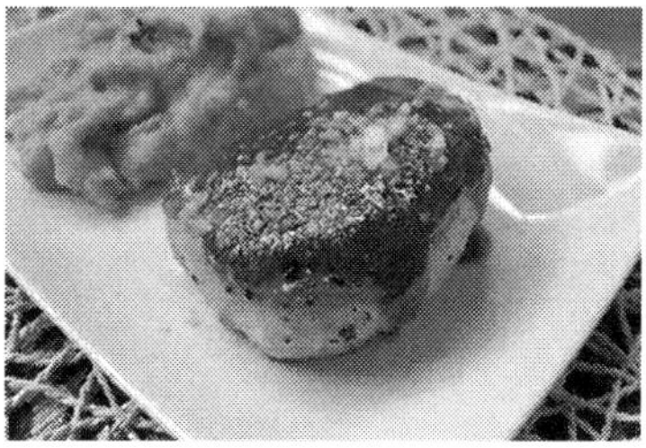

Pesto Pork Chops

Prep time: 20 minutes	Cook time: 20 minutes	Servings: 4

Ingredients

- Pork top-loin chops – 4 (3-ounce) boneless, fat trimmed
- Herb pesto – 8 tsps.
- Breadcrumbs – ½ cup
- Olive oil – 1 Tbsp.

Method

1. Preheat the oven to 450F.
2. Line a baking sheet with foil. Set aside.
3. Rub 1 tsp. of pesto evenly over both sides of each pork chop.
4. Lightly dredge each pork chop in the breadcrumbs.
5. Heat the oil in a skillet.
6. Brown the pork chops on each side for 5 minutes.
7. Place the pork chops on the baking sheet.
8. Bake for 10 minutes or until pork reaches 145F in the center.

Nutritional Facts Per Serving

- Calories: 210

- Fat: 7g
- Carb: 10g
- Phosphorus: 179mg
- Potassium: 220mg
- Sodium: 148mg
- Protein: 24g

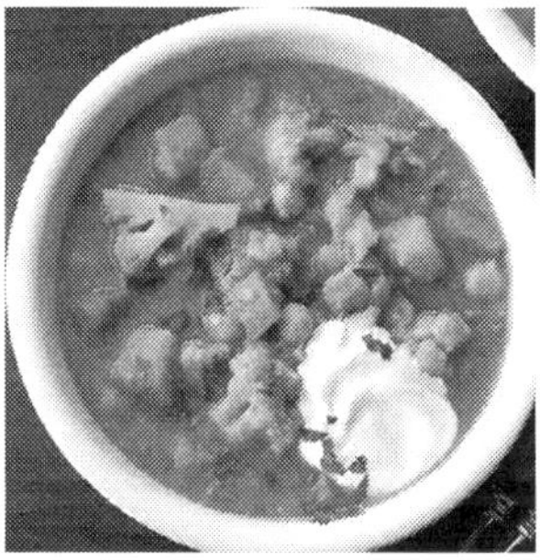

Vegetable Curry

Prep time: 15 minutes	Cook time: 45 minutes	Servings: 4

Ingredients

- Olive oil – 2 tsps.
- Sweet onion – ½, diced
- Minced garlic – 2 tsps.
- Grated fresh ginger – 2 tsps.
- Eggplant – ½, peeled and diced
- Carrot – 1, peeled and diced
- Red bell pepper – 1, diced

- Hot curry powder – 1 Tbsp.
- Ground cumin – 1 tsp.
- Coriander – ½ tsp.
- Pinch cayenne pepper
- Homemade vegetable stock – 1 ½ cups
- Cornstarch – 1 Tbsp.
- Water – ¼ cup

Method

1. Heat the oil in a stockpot.
2. Sauté the ginger, garlic, and onion for 3 minutes or until they are softened.
3. Add the red pepper, carrots, eggplant, and stir often for 6 minutes.
4. Stir in the cumin, curry powder, coriander, cayenne pepper, and vegetable stock.
5. Bring the curry to a boil and then lower the heat to low.
6. Simmer the curry for 30 minutes or until the vegetables are tender.
7. In a bowl, stir together the cornstarch and water.
8. Stir in the cornstarch mixture into the curry and simmer for 5 minutes or until the sauce has thickened.

Nutritional Facts Per Serving

- Calories: 100
- Fat: 3g
- Carb: 9g

- Phosphorus: 28mg
- Potassium: 180mg
- Sodium: 218mg
- Protein: 1g

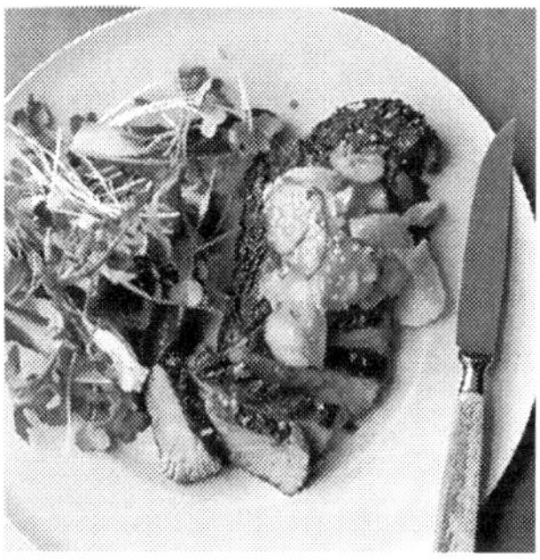

Grilled Steak with Salsa

Prep time: 20 minutes	Cook time: 15 minutes	Servings: 4

Ingredients for the salsa

- Chopped English cucumber - 1 cup
- Boiled and diced red bell pepper – ¼ cup
- Scallion – 1, both green and white parts, chopped
- Chopped fresh cilantro – 2 Tbsps.
- Juice of 1 lime

For the steak

- Beef tenderloin steaks – 4 (3-ounce), room temperature
- Olive oil
- Freshly ground black pepper

Method

1. To make the salsa, in a bowl, combine the lime juice, cilantro, scallion, bell pepper, and cucumber. Set aside.
2. To make the steak: Preheat a barbecue to medium heat.
3. Rub the steaks all over with oil and season with pepper.
4. Grill the steaks for about 5 minutes per side for medium-rare, or until the desired doneness.
5. Serve the steaks topped with salsa.

Nutritional Facts Per Serving

- Calories: 130
- Fat: 6g
- Carb: 1g
- Phosphorus: 186mg
- Potassium: 272mg
- Sodium: 39mg
- Protein: 19g

Chapter 7 Dinner Recipes

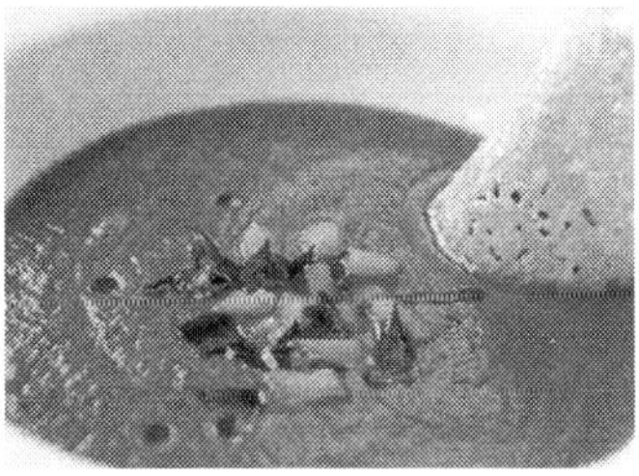

Eggplant and Red Pepper Soup

Prep time: 20 minutes	Cook time: 40 minutes	Servings: 6

Ingredients

- Sweet onion – 1 small, cut into quarters
- Small red bell peppers – 2, halved
- Cubed eggplant – 2 cups
- Garlic – 2 cloves, crushed
- Olive oil – 1 Tbsp.
- Chicken stock – 1 cup
- Water
- Chopped fresh basil – ¼ cup
- Ground black pepper

Method

1. Preheat the oven to 350F.
2. Put the onions, red peppers, eggplant, and garlic in a baking dish.

3. Drizzle the vegetables with the olive oil.
4. Roast the vegetables for 30 minutes or until they are slightly charred and soft.
5. Cool the vegetables slightly and remove the skin from the peppers.
6. Puree the vegetables with a hand mixer (with the chicken stock).
7. Transfer the soup to a medium pot and add enough water to reach the desired thickness.
8. Heat the soup to a simmer and add the basil.
9. Season with pepper and serve.

Nutritional Facts Per Serving

- Calories: 61
- Fat: 2g
- Carb: 9g
- Phosphorus: 33mg
- Potassium: 198mg
- Sodium: 98mg
- Protein: 2g

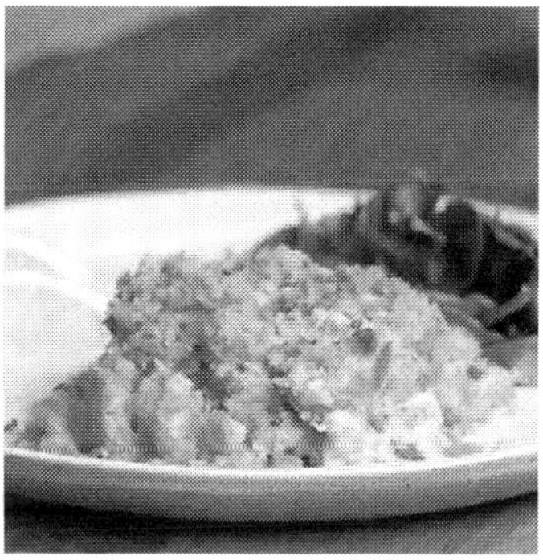

Seafood Casserole

Prep time: 20 minutes	Cook time: 45 minutes	Servings: 6

Ingredients

- Eggplant – 2 cups, peeled and diced into 1-inch pieces
- Butter, for greasing the baking dish
- Olive oil – 1 tbsp.
- Sweet onion – ½, chopped
- Minced garlic - 1 tsp.
- Celery stalk – 1, chopped
- Red bell pepper – ½, boiled and chopped
- Freshly squeezed lemon juice – 3 Tbsps.
- Hot sauce – 1 tsp.
- Creole seasoning mix – ¼ tsp.
- White rice – ½ cup, uncooked
- Egg – 1 large

- Cooked shrimp – 4 ounces
- Queen crab meat – 6 ounces

Method

1. Preheat the oven to 350F.
2. Boil the eggplant in a saucepan for 5 minutes. Drain and set aside.
3. Grease a 9-by-13-inch baking dish with butter and set aside.
4. Heat the olive oil in a large skillet over medium heat.
5. Sauté the garlic, onion, celery, and bell pepper for 4 minutes or until tender.
6. Add the sautéed vegetables to the eggplant, along with the lemon juice, hot sauce, seasoning, rice, and egg.
7. Stir to combine.
8. Fold in the shrimp and crab meat.
9. Spoon the casserole mixture into the casserole dish, patting down the top.
10. Bake for 25 to 30 minutes or until casserole is heated through and rice is tender.
11. Serve warm.

Nutritional Facts Per Serving

- Calories: 118
- Fat: 4g
- Carb: 9g
- Phosphorus: 102mg
- Potassium: 199mg
- Sodium: 235mg

- Protein: 12g

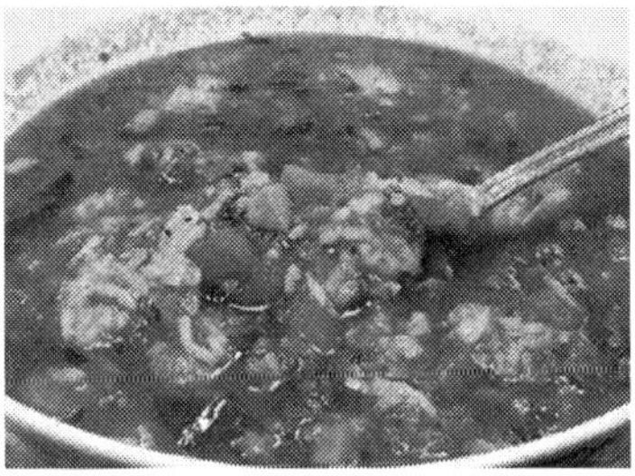

Ground Beef and Rice Soup

Prep time: 15 minutes	Cook time: 40 minutes	Servings: 6

Ingredients

- Extra-lean ground beef – ½ pound
- Small sweet onion – ½, chopped
- Minced garlic – 1 tsp.
- Water – 2 cups
- Low-sodium beef broth – 1 cup
- Long-grain white rice – ½ cup, uncooked
- Celery stalk – 1, chopped
- Fresh green beans – ½ cup, cut into – 1-inch pieces
- Chopped fresh thyme – 1 tsp.
- Ground black pepper

Method

1. Sauté the ground beef in a saucepan for 6 minutes or until the beef is completely browned.

2. Drain off the excess fat and add the onion and garlic to the saucepan.
3. Sauté the vegetables for about 3 minutes, or until they are softened.
4. Add the celery, rice, beef broth, and water.
5. Bring the soup to a boil, reduce the heat to low and simmer for 30 minutes or until the rice is tender.
6. Add the green beans and thyme and simmer for 3 minutes.
7. Remove the soup from the heat and season with pepper.

Nutritional Facts Per Serving

- Calories: 154
- Fat: 7g
- Carb: 14g
- Phosphorus: 76mg
- Potassium: 179mg
- Sodium: 133mg
- Protein: 9g

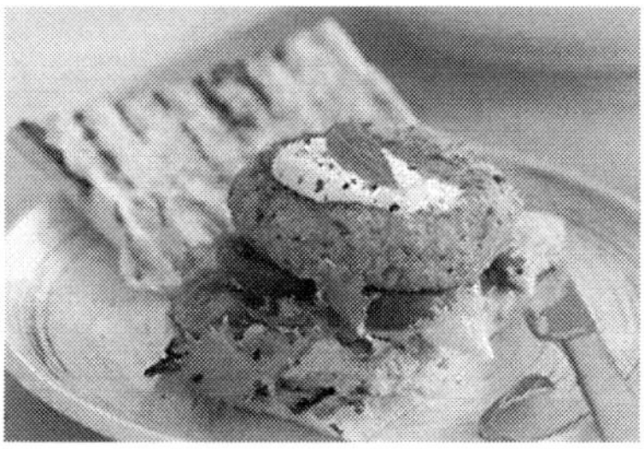

Couscous Burgers

Prep time: 20 minutes	Cook time: 10 minutes	Servings: 4

Ingredients

- Canned chickpeas – ½ cup, rinsed and drained
- Chopped fresh cilantro – 2 Tbsps.
- Chopped fresh parsley
- Lemon juice - 1 Tbsp.
- Lemon zest – 2 tsps.
- Minced garlic – 1 tsp.
- Cooked couscous – 2 ½ cups
- Eggs – 2 lightly beaten
- Olive oil – 2 Tbsps.

Method

1. Put the cilantro, chickpeas, parsley, lemon juice, lemon zest, and garlic in a food processor and pulse until a paste forms.
2. Transfer the chickpea mixture to a bowl and add the eggs and couscous. Mix well.
3. Chill the mixture in the refrigerator for 1 hour.
4. Form the couscous mixture into 4 patties.
5. Heat olive oil in a skillet.
6. Place the patties in the skillet, 2 at a time, gently pressing them down with a spatula.
7. Cook for 5 minutes or until golden and flip the patties over.
8. Cook the other side for 5 minutes and transfer the cooked burgers to a plate covered with a paper towel.
9. Repeat with the remaining 2 burgers.

Nutritional Facts Per Serving

- Calories: 242
- Fat: 10g
- Carb: 29g
- Phosphorus: 108mg
- Potassium: 168mg
- Sodium: 43mg
- Protein: 9g

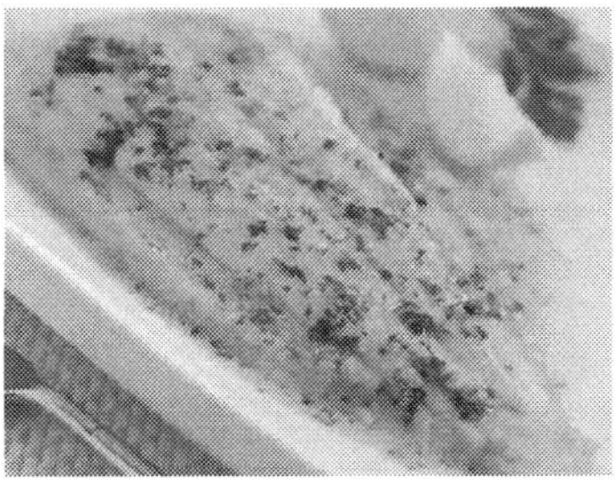

Baked Flounder

Prep time: 20 minutes	Cook time: 5 minutes	Servings: 4

Ingredients

- Homemade mayonnaise – ¼ cup
- Juice of 1 lime
- Zest of 1 lime
- Chopped fresh cilantro – ½ cup
- Flounder fillets – 4 (3-ounce)

- Ground black pepper

Method

1. Preheat the oven to 400F.
2. In a bowl, stir together the cilantro, lime juice, lime zest, and mayonnaise.
3. Place 4 pieces of foil, about 8 by 8 inches square, on a clean work surface.
4. Place a flounder fillet in the center of each square.
5. Top the fillets evenly with the mayonnaise mixture.
6. Season the flounder with pepper.
7. Fold the sides of the foil over the fish, creating a snug packet, and place the foil packets on a baking sheet.
8. Bake the fish for 4 to 5 minutes.
9. Unfold the packets and serve.

Nutritional Facts Per Serving

- Calories: 92
- Fat: 4g
- Carb: 2g
- Phosphorus: 208mg
- Potassium: 137mg
- Sodium: 267mg
- Protein: 12g

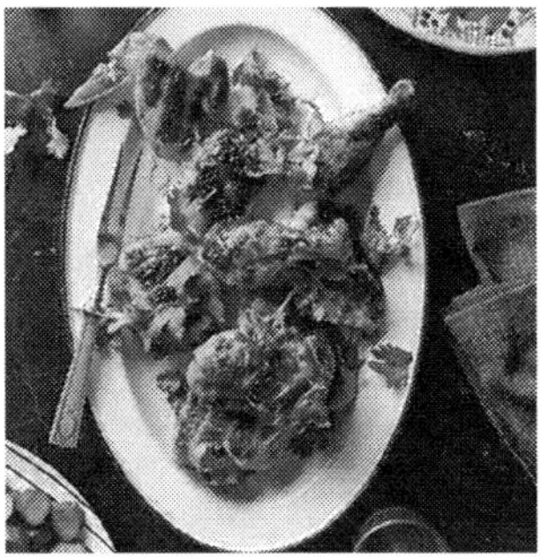

Persian Chicken

Prep time: 10 minutes	Cook time: 20 minutes	Servings: 5

Ingredients

- Sweet onion – ½, chopped
- Lemon juice – ¼ cup
- Dried oregano – 1 Tbsp.
- Minced garlic – 1 tsp.
- Sweet paprika – 1 tsp.
- Ground cumin – ½ tsp.
- Olive oil – ½ cup
- Boneless, skinless chicken thighs – 5

Method

1. Put the cumin, paprika, garlic, oregano, lemon juice, and onion in a food processor and pulse to mix the ingredients.
2. Keep the motor running and add the olive oil until the mixture is smooth.

3. Place the chicken thighs in a large sealable freezer bag and pour the marinade into the bag.
4. Seal the bag and place in the refrigerator, turning the bag twice, for 2 hours.
5. Remove the thighs from the marinade and discard the extra marinade.
6. Preheat the barbecue to medium.
7. Grill the chicken for about 20 minutes, turning once, until it reaches 165F.

Nutritional Facts Per Serving

- Calories: 321
- Fat: 21g
- Carb: 3g
- Phosphorus: 131mg
- Potassium: 220mg
- Sodium: 86mg
- Protein: 22g

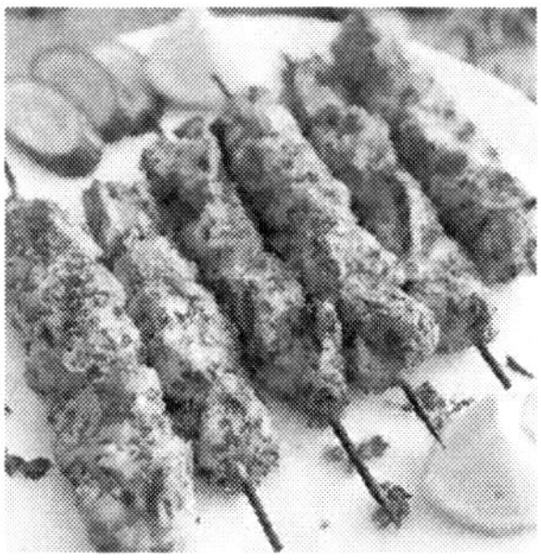

Pork Souvlaki

Prep time: 20 minutes	Cook time: 12 minutes	Servings: 8

Ingredients

- Olive oil – 3 Tbsps.
- Lemon juice – 2 Tbsps.
- Minced garlic – 1 tsp.
- Chopped fresh oregano – 1 Tbsp.
- Ground black pepper – ¼ tsp.
- Pork leg – 1 pound, cut in 2-inch cubes

Method

1. In a bowl, stir together the lemon juice, olive oil, garlic, oregano, and pepper.
2. Add the pork cubes and toss to coat.
3. Place the bowl in the refrigerator, covered, for 2 hours to marinate.
4. Thread the pork chunks onto 8 wooden skewers that have been soaked in water.
5. Preheat the barbecue to medium-high heat.
6. Grill the pork skewers for about 12 minutes, turning once, until just cooked through but still juicy.

Nutritional Facts Per Serving

- Calories: 95
- Fat: 4g
- Carb: 0g
- Phosphorus: 125mg
- Potassium: 230mg

- Sodium: 29mg
- Protein: 13g

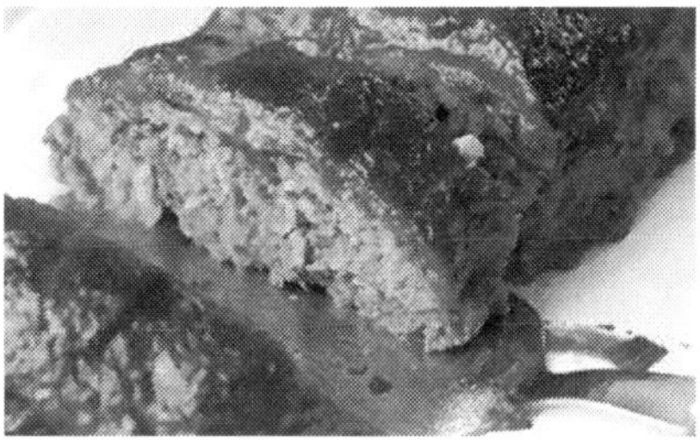

Pork Meatloaf

Prep time: 10 minutes	Cook time: 50 minutes	Servings: 8

Ingredients

- 95% lean ground beef – 1 pound
- Breadcrumbs – ½ cup
- Chopped sweet onion – ½ cup
- Egg – 1
- Chopped fresh basil – 2 Tbsps.
- Chopped fresh thyme -1 tsp.
- Chopped fresh parsley – 1 tsp.
- Ground black pepper – ¼ tsp.
- Brown sugar – 1 Tbsp.
- White vinegar – 1 tsp.
- Garlic powder – ¼ tsp.

Method

1. Preheat the oven to 350F.
2. Mix together the breadcrumbs, beef, onion, basil, egg, thyme, parsley, and pepper until well combined.
3. Press the meat mixture into a 9-by-5-inch loaf pan.
4. In a small bowl, stir together the brown sugar, vinegar, and garlic powder.
5. Spread the brown sugar mixture evenly over the meat.
6. Bake the meatloaf for about 50 minutes or until it is cooked through.
7. Let the meatloaf stand for 10 minutes and then pour out any accumulated grease.

Nutritional Facts Per Serving

- Calories: 103
- Fat: 3g
- Carb: 7g
- Phosphorus: 112mg
- Potassium: 190mg
- Sodium: 87mg
- Protein: 11g

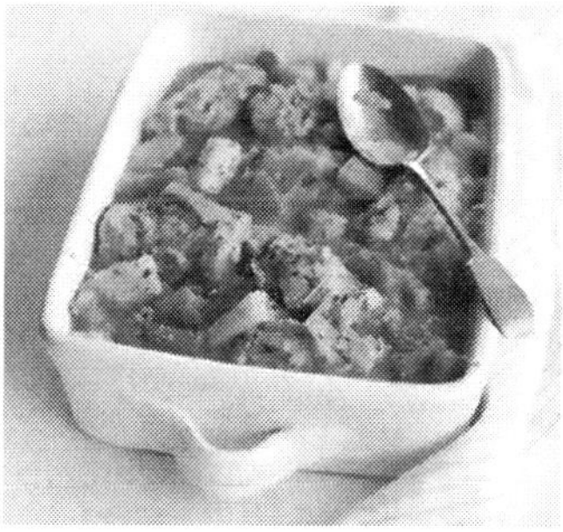

Chicken Stew

Prep time: 20 minutes	Cook time: 50 minutes	Servings: 6

Ingredients

- Olive oil – 1 Tbsp.
- Boneless, skinless chicken thighs – 1 pound, cut into 1-inch cubes
- Sweet onion – ½, chopped
- Minced garlic – 1 Tbsp.
- Chicken stock – 2 cups
- Water – 1 cup, plus 2 Tbsps.
- Carrot – 1, sliced
- Celery – 2 stalks, sliced
- Turnip – 1, sliced thin
- Chopped fresh thyme – 1 Tbsp.
- Chopped fresh rosemary – 1 tsp.
- Cornstarch – 2 tsps.

- Ground black pepper to taste

Method

1. Place a large saucepan on medium heat and add the olive oil.
2. Sauté the chicken for 6 minutes or until it is lightly browned, stirring often.
3. Add the onion and garlic, and sauté for 3 minutes.
4. Add 1-cup water, chicken stock, carrot, celery, and turnip and bring the stew to a boil.
5. Reduce the heat to low and simmer for 30 minutes or until the chicken is cooked through and tender.
6. Add the thyme and rosemary and simmer for 3 minutes more.
7. In a small bowl, stir together the 2 tbsps. Of water and the cornstarch; add the mixture to the stew.
8. Stir to incorporate the cornstarch mixture and cook for 3 to 4 minutes or until the stew thickens.
9. Remove from the heat and season with pepper.

Nutritional Facts Per Serving

- Calories: 141
- Fat: 8g
- Carb: 5g
- Phosphorus: 53mg
- Potassium: 192mg
- Sodium: 214mg
- Protein: 9g

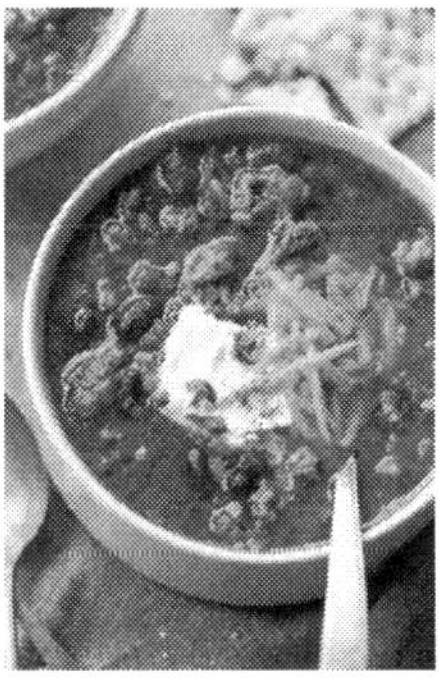

Beef Chili

Prep time: 10 minutes	Cook time: 30 minutes	Servings: 2

Ingredients

- Onion – 1, diced
- Red bell pepper – 1, diced
- Garlic – 2 cloves, minced
- Lean ground beef – 6 oz.
- Chili powder – 1 tsp.
- Oregano – 1 tsp.
- Extra virgin olive oil – 2 Tbsps.
- Water – 1 cup
- Brown rice -1 cup
- Fresh cilantro – 1 Tbsp. to serve

Method

1. Soak vegetables in warm water.

2. Bring a pan of water to the boil and add rice for 20 minutes.
3. Meanwhile, add the oil to a pan and heat on medium-high heat.
4. Add the pepper, onions, and garlic and sauté for 5 minutes until soft.
5. Remove and set aside.
6. Add the beef to the pan and stir until browned.
7. Add the vegetables back into the pan and stir.
8. Now add the chili powder and herbs and the water, cover and turn the heat down a little to simmer for 15 minutes.
9. Meanwhile, drain the water from the rice, and the lid and steam while the chili is cooking.
10. Serve hot with the fresh cilantro sprinkled over the top.

Nutritional Facts Per Serving

- Calories: 459
- Fat: 22g
- Carb: 36g
- Phosphorus: 332mg
- Potassium: 360mg
- Sodium: 33mg
- Protein: 22g

Chapter 8 Snacks & Side Dishes

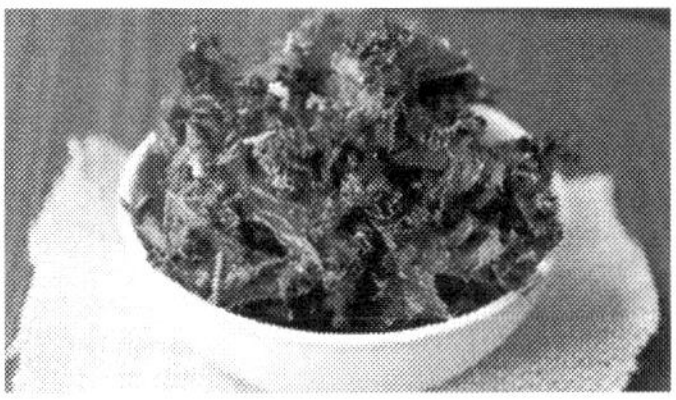

Kale Chips

Prep time: 20 minutes	Cook time: 25 minutes	Servings: 6

Ingredients

- Kale – 2 cups
- Olive oil – 2 tsp.
- Chili powder – ¼ tsp.
- Pinch cayenne pepper

Method

1. Preheat the oven to 300F.
2. Line 2 baking sheets with parchment paper; set aside.
3. Remove the stems from the kale and tear the leaves into 2-inch pieces.
4. Wash the kale and dry it completely.
5. Transfer the kale to a large bowl and drizzle with olive oil.
6. Use your hands to toss the kale with oil, taking care to coat each leaf evenly.
7. Season the kale with chili powder and cayenne pepper and toss to combine thoroughly.
8. Spread the seasoned kale in a single layer on each baking sheet. Do not overlap the leaves.

9. Bake the kale, rotating the pans once, for 20 to 25 minutes until it is crisp and dry.
10. Remove the trays from the oven and allow the chips to cool on the trays for 5 minutes.
11. Serve.

Nutritional Facts Per Serving

- Calories: 24
- Fat: 2g
- Carb: 2g
- Phosphorus: 21mg
- Potassium: 111mg
- Sodium: 13mg
- Protein: 1g

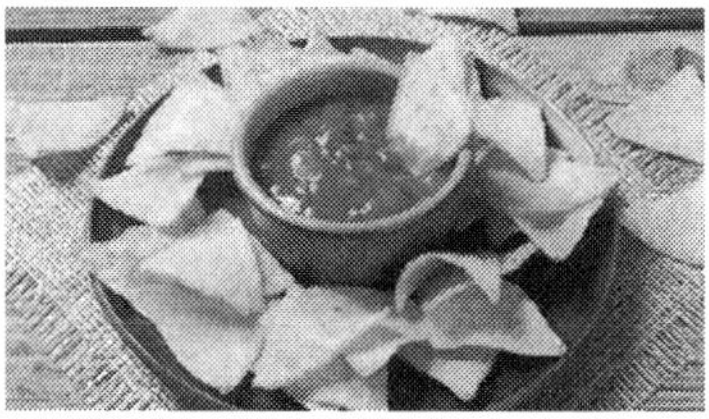

Tortilla Chips

Prep time: 15 minutes	Cook time: 10 minutes	Servings: 6

Ingredients

- Granulated sugar – 2 tsps.
- Ground cinnamon – ½ tsp.
- Pinch ground nutmeg

- Flour tortillas – 3 (6-inch)
- Cooking spray

Method

1. Preheat the oven to 350F.
2. Line a baking sheet with parchment paper.
3. In a small bowl, stir together the sugar, cinnamon, and nutmeg.
4. Lay the tortillas on a clean work surface and spray both sides of each lightly with cooking spray.
5. Sprinkle the cinnamon sugar evenly over both sides of each tortilla.
6. Cut the tortillas into 16 wedges each and place them on the baking sheet.
7. Bake the tortilla wedges, turning once, for about 10 minutes or until crisp.
8. Cool the chips serve.

Nutritional Facts Per Serving

- Calories: 51
- Fat: 1g
- Carb: 9g
- Phosphorus: 29mg
- Potassium: 24mg
- Sodium:103 mg
- Protein: 1g

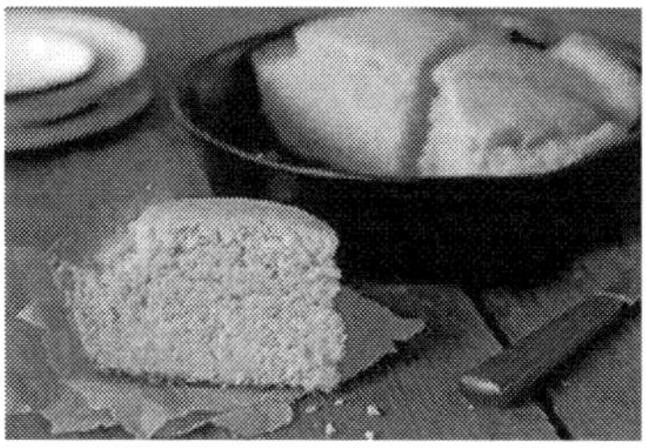

Corn Bread

Prep time: 10 minutes	Cook time: 20 minutes	Servings: 10

Ingredients

- Cooking spray for greasing the baking dish
- Yellow cornmeal – 1 ¼ cups
- All-purpose flour – ¾ cup
- Baking soda substitute – 1 tbsp.
- Granulated sugar – ½ cup
- Eggs – 2
- Unsweetened, unfortified rice milk – 1 cup
- Olive oil – 2 Tbsps.

Method

1. Preheat the oven to 425F.
2. Lightly spray an 8-by-8-inch baking dish with cooking spray. Set aside.
3. In a medium bowl, stir together the cornmeal, flour, baking soda substitute, and sugar.
4. In a small bowl, whisk together the eggs, rice milk, and olive oil until blended.

5. Add the wet ingredients to the dry ingredients and stir until well combined.
6. Pour the batter into the baking dish and bake for 20 minutes or until golden and cooked through.
7. Serve warm.

Nutritional Facts Per Serving

- Calories: 198
- Fat: 5g
- Carb: 34g
- Phosphorus: 88mg
- Potassium: 94mg
- Sodium: 25mg
- Protein: 4g

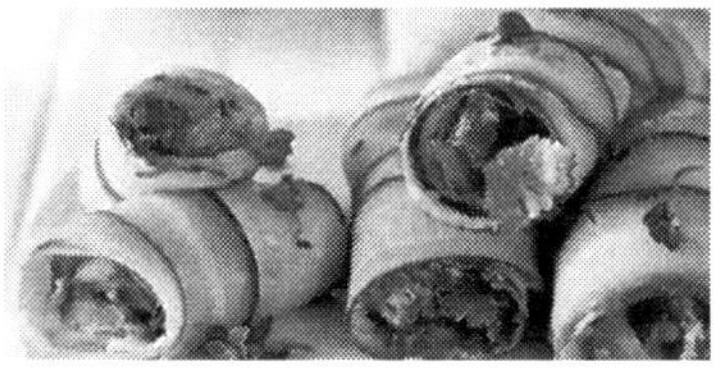

Vegetable Rolls

Prep time: 30 minutes	Cook time: 0 minutes	Servings: 8

Ingredients

- Finely shredded red cabbage – ½ cup
- Grated carrot – ½ cup
- Julienne red bell pepper – ¼ cup

- Julienned scallion – ¼ cup, both green and white parts
- Chopped cilantro – ¼ cup
- Olive oil – 1 Tbsp.
- Ground cumin – ¼ tsp.
- Freshly ground black pepper – ¼ tsp.
- English cucumber – 1, sliced very thin strips

Method

1. In a bowl, toss together the black pepper, cumin, olive oil, cilantro, scallion, red pepper, carrot, and cabbage. Mix well.
2. Evenly divide the vegetable filling among the cucumber strips, placing the filling close to one end of the strip.
3. Roll up the cucumber strips around the filling and secure with a wooden pick.
4. Repeat with each cucumber strip.

Nutritional Facts Per Serving

- Calories: 26
- Fat: 2g
- Carb: 3g
- Phosphorus: 14mg
- Potassium: 95mg
- Sodium: 7mg
- Protein: 0g

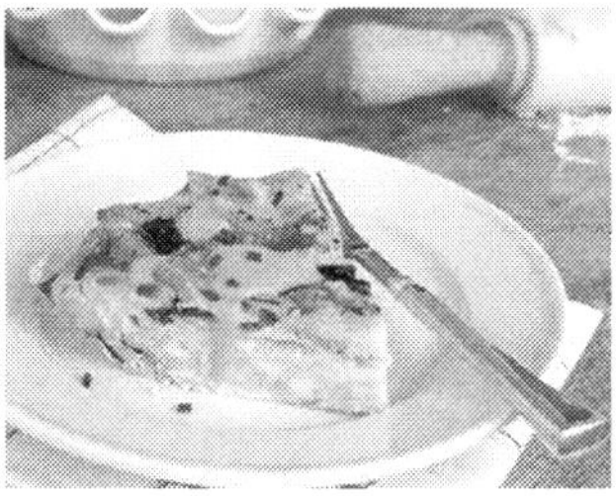

Frittata with Penne

Prep time: 15 minutes	Cook time: 30 minutes	Servings: 4

Ingredients

- Egg whites- 6
- Rice milk – ¼ cup
- Chopped fresh parsley – 1 Tbsp.
- Chopped fresh thyme – 1 tsp.
- Chopped fresh chives – 1 tsp.
- Ground black pepper
- Olive oil – 2 tsps.
- Small sweet onion – ¼, chopped
- Minced garlic – 1 tsp.
- Boiled and chopped red bell pepper – ½ cup
- Cooked penne – 2 cups

Method

1. Preheat the oven to 350F.

2. In a bowl, whisk together the egg whites, rice milk, parsley, thyme, chives, and pepper.
3. Heat the oil in a skillet.
4. Sauté the onion, garlic, red pepper for 4 minutes or until they are softened.
5. Add the cooked penne to the skillet.
6. Pour the egg mixture over the pasta and shake the pan to coat the pasta.
7. Leave the skillet on the heat for 1 minute to set the bottom of the frittata and then transfer the skillet to the oven.
8. Bake, the frittata for 25 minutes or until it is set and golden brown.
9. Serve.

Nutritional Facts Per Serving

- Calories: 170
- Fat: 3g
- Carb: 25g
- Phosphorus: 62mg
- Potassium: 144mg
- Sodium: 90mg
- Protein: 10g

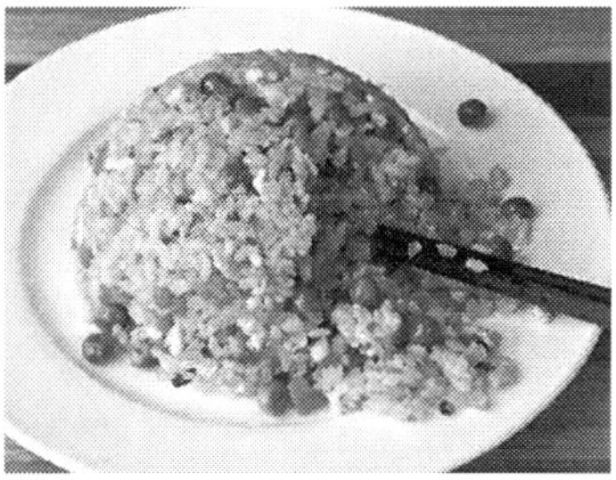

Vegetable Fried Rice

Prep time: 20 minutes	Cook time: 20 minutes	Servings: 6

Ingredients

- Olive oil – 1 Tbsp.
- Sweet onion – ½, chopped
- Grated fresh ginger – 1 Tbsp.
- Minced garlic - 2 tsps.
- Sliced carrots – 1 cup
- Chopped eggplant – ½ cup
- Peas – ½ cup
- Green beans – ½ cup, cut into 1-inch pieces
- Chopped fresh cilantro – 2 Tbsp.
- Cooked rice – 3 cups

Method

1. Heat the olive oil in a skillet.
2. Sauté the ginger, onion, and garlic for 3 minutes or until softened.

3. Stir in carrot, eggplant, green beans, and peas and sauté for 3 minutes more.
4. Add cilantro and rice.
5. Sauté, constantly stirring, for about 10 minutes or until the rice is heated through.
6. Serve.

Nutritional Facts Per Serving

- Calories: 189
- Fat: 7g
- Carb: 28g
- Phosphorus: 89mg
- Potassium: 172mg
- Sodium: 13mg
- Protein: 6g

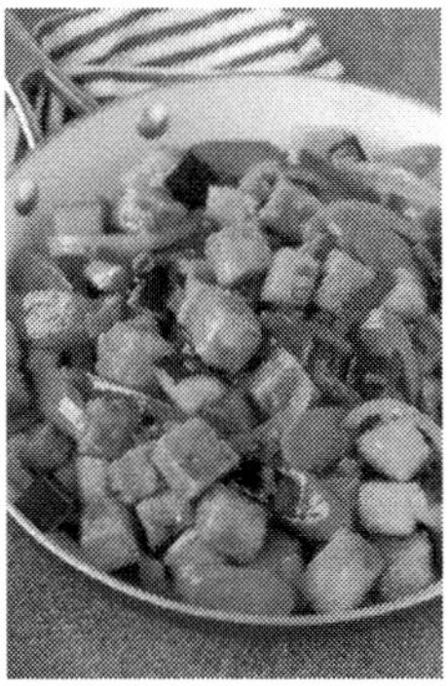

Tofu Stir-Fry

Prep time: 20 minutes	Cook time: 20 minutes	Servings: 4

Ingredients for the tofu

- Lemon juice – 1 Tbsp.
- Minced garlic – 1 tsp.
- Grated fresh ginger – 1 tsp.
- Pinch red pepper flakes
- Extra-firm tofu- 5 ounces, pressed well and cubed

For the stir-fry

- Olive oil – 1 Tbsp.
- Cauliflower florets – ½ cup
- Thinly sliced carrots – ½ cup
- Julienned red pepper – ½ cup
- Fresh green beans – ½ cup
- Cooked white rice – 2 cups

Method

1. In a bowl, mix the lemon juice, garlic, ginger, and red pepper flakes.
2. Add the tofu and toss to coat.
3. Place the bowl in the refrigerator and marinate for 2 hours.
4. To make the stir-fry, heat the oil in a skillet.
5. Sauté the tofu for 8 minutes or until it is lightly browned and heated through.
6. Add the carrots, and cauliflower and sauté for 5 minutes. Stirring and tossing constantly.
7. Add the red pepper and green beans, sauté for 3 minutes more.
8. Serve over white rice.

Nutritional Facts Per Serving

- Calories: 190
- Fat: 6g
- Carb: 30g
- Phosphorus: 90mg
- Potassium: 199mg
- Sodium: 22mg
- Protein: 6g

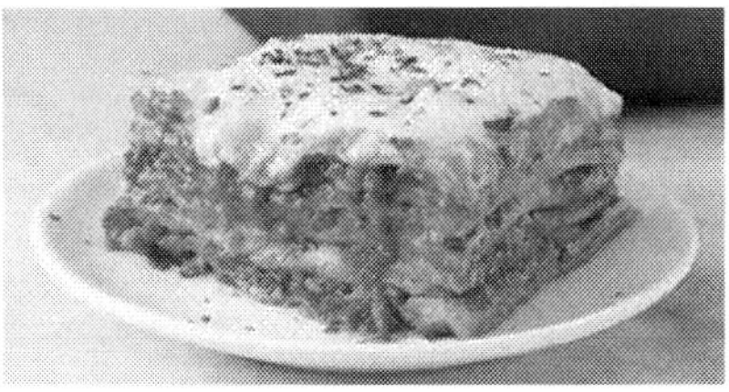

Lasagna

Prep time: 10 minutes	Cook time: 1 hour	Servings: 2

Ingredients

- Soft tofu - ½ pack
- Baby spinach – ½ cup
- Unenriched rick milk – 4 Tbsps.
- Garlic – 1 clove, crushed
- Lemon – 1, juiced
- Fresh basil – 2 Tbsps. chopped
- A pinch of black pepper to taste

- Zucchini – 1, sliced
- Red bell pepper – 1, sliced
- Eggplant – 1 sliced

Method

1. Preheat the oven to 325F. Soak vegetables in warm water prior to cooking.
2. In a blender, process the tofu, garlic, milk, basil, lemon juice, and pepper until smooth.
3. Toss in the zucchini and spinach for the last 30 seconds.
4. Layer the bottom of the dish with 1/3 eggplant slices and 1/3 red pepper slices and then cover with 1/3 of the tofu sauce. Repeat to complete.
5. Bake in the oven for 1 hour or until the vegetables are soft through to the center.
6. Finish under the broiler until golden and bubbly.
7. Divide into portions and serve with a sprinkle of black pepper to taste.

Nutritional Facts Per Serving

- Calories: 116
- Fat: 4g
- Carb: 10g
- Phosphorus: 149mg
- Potassium: 346mg
- Sodium: 27mg
- Protein: 5g

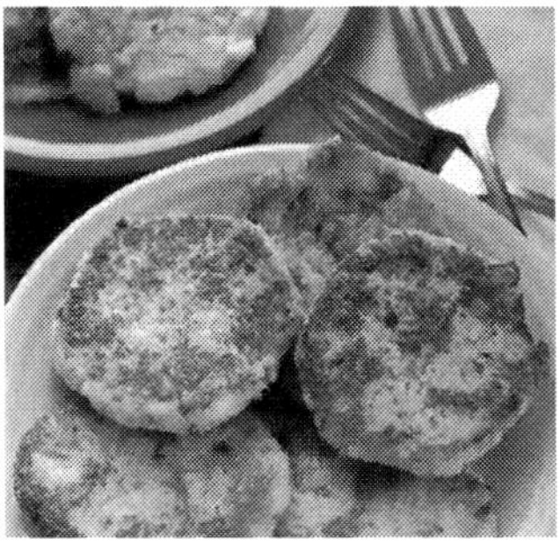

Cauliflower Patties

Prep time: 5 minutes	Cook time: 8 minutes	Servings: 2

Ingredients

- Eggs – 2
- Egg whites – 2
- Onion – ½, diced
- Cauliflower – 2 cups, frozen
- All-purpose white flour – 2 Tbsps.
- Black pepper – 1 tsp.
- Coconut oil – 1 Tbsp.
- Curry powder – 1 tsp.
- Fresh cilantro – 1 Tbsp.

Method

1. Soak vegetables in warm water prior to cooking.
2. Steam cauliflower over a pan of boiling water for 10 minutes.

3. Blend eggs and onion in a food processor before adding cooked cauliflower, spices, cilantro, flour, and pepper and blast in the processor for 30 seconds.
4. Heat a skillet on a high heat and add oil.
5. Pour tbsp. portions of the cauliflower mixture into the pan and brown on each side until crispy, about 3 to 4 minutes.
6. Enjoy with a salad.

Nutritional Facts Per Serving

- Calories: 227
- Fat: 12g
- Carb: 15g
- Phosphorus: 193mg
- Potassium: 513mg
- Sodium: 158mg
- Protein: 13g

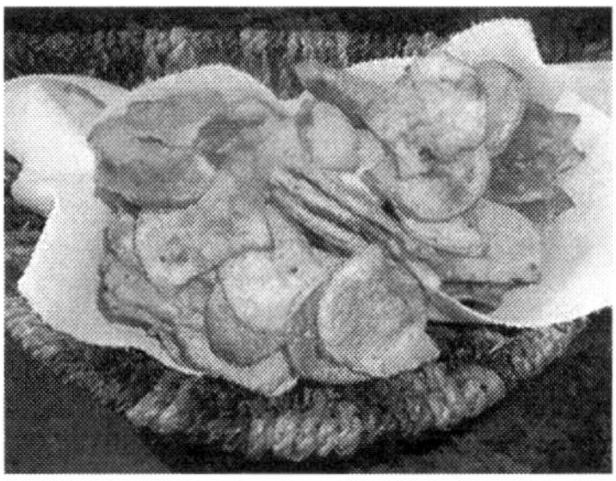

Turnip Chips

Prep time: 5 minutes	Cook time: 50 minutes	Servings: 2

Ingredients

- Turnips – 2, peeled and sliced
- Extra virgin olive oil – 1 Tbsp.
- Onion – 1 chopped
- Minced garlic – 1 clove
- Black pepper – 1 tsp.
- Oregano – 1 tsp.
- Paprika - 1 1 tsp.

Method

1. Preheat oven to 375F. Grease a baking tray with olive oil.
2. Add turnip slices in a thin layer.
3. Dust over herbs and spices with an extra drizzle of olive oil.
4. Bake 40 minutes. Turning once.

Nutritional Facts Per Serving

- Calories: 136
- Fat: 14g
- Carb: 30g
- Phosphorus: 50mg
- Potassium: 356mg
- Sodium: 71mg
- Protein: g

Chapter 9 Desserts

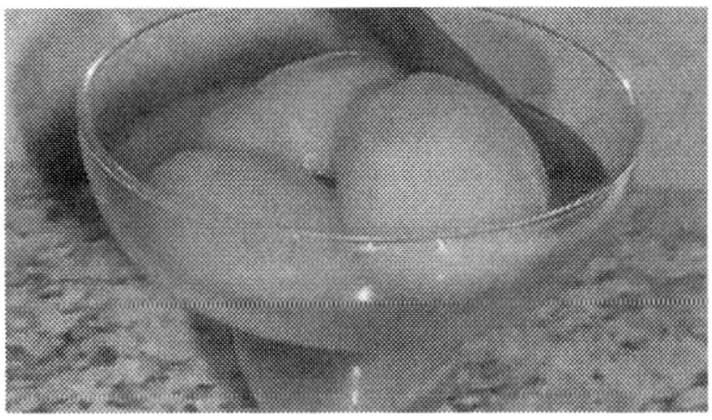

Spiced Peaches

Prep time: 5 minutes	Cook time: 10 minutes	Servings: 2

Ingredients

- Canned peaches with juices – 1 cup
- Cornstarch – ½ tsp.
- Ground cloves – 1 tsp.
- Ground cinnamon – 1 tsp.
- Ground nutmeg – 1 tsp.
- Zest of ½ lemon
- Water – ½ cup

Method

1. Drain peaches.
2. Combine cinnamon, cornstarch, nutmeg, ground cloves, and lemon zest in a pan on the stove.
3. Heat on a medium heat and add peaches.
4. Bring to a boil, reduce the heat and simmer for 10 minutes.
5. Serve.

Nutritional Facts Per Serving

- Calories: 70
- Fat: 0g
- Carb: 14g
- Phosphorus: 23mg
- Potassium: 176mg
- Sodium: 3mg
- Protein: 1g

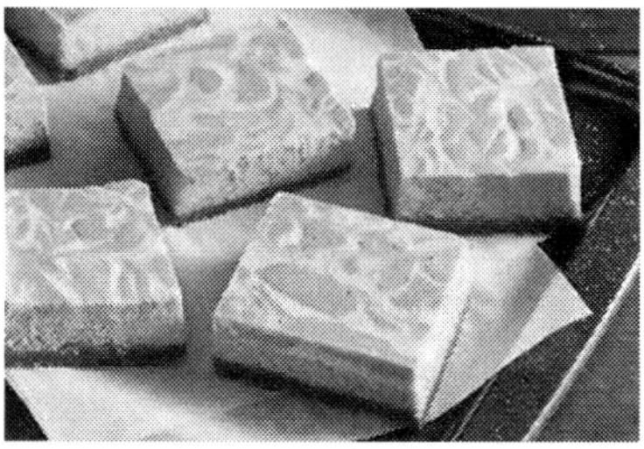

Pumpkin Cheesecake Bar

Prep time: 10 minutes	Cook time: 50 minutes	Servings: 4

Ingredients

- Unsalted butter – 2 ½ Tbsps.
- Cream cheese – 4 oz.
- All-purpose white flour – ½ cup
- Golden brown sugar – 3 Tbsps.
- Granulated sugar – ¼ cup
- Pureed pumpkin – ½ cup

- Egg whites - 2
- Ground cinnamon – 1 tsp.
- Ground nutmeg – 1 tsp.
- Vanilla extract – 1 tsp.

Method

1. Preheat the oven to 350F.
2. Mix flour and brown sugar in a bowl.
3. Mix in the butter to form 'breadcrumbs'.
4. Place ¾ of this mixture in a dish.
5. Bake in the oven for 15 minutes. Remove and cool.
6. Lightly whisk the egg and fold in the cream cheese, sugar, pumpkin, cinnamon, nutmeg and vanilla until smooth.
7. Pour this mixture over the oven-baked base and sprinkle with the rest of the breadcrumbs from earlier.
8. Bake in the oven for 30 to 35 minutes more.
9. Cool, slice and serve.

Nutritional Facts Per Serving

- Calories: 248
- Fat: 13g
- Carb: 33g
- Phosphorus: 67mg
- Potassium: 96mg
- Sodium: 146mg
- Protein: 4g

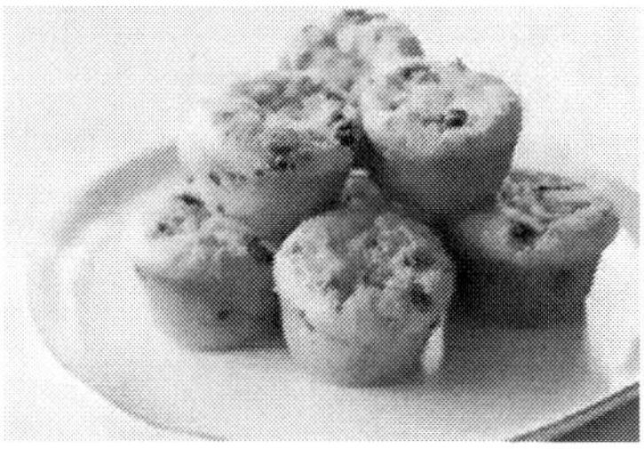

Blueberry Mini Muffins

Prep time: 10 minutes	Cook time: 35 minutes	Servings: 4

Ingredients

- Egg whites – 3
- All-purpose white flour – ¼ cup
- Coconut flour – 1 Tbsp.
- Baking soda – 1 tsp.
- Nutmeg – 1 Tbsp. grated
- Vanilla extract – 1 tsp.
- Stevia – 1 tsp.
- Fresh blueberries – ¼ cup

Method

1. Preheat the oven to 325F.
2. Mix all the ingredients in a bowl.
3. Divide the batter into 4 and spoon into a lightly oiled muffin tin.
4. Bake in the oven for 15 to 20 minutes or until cooked through.
5. Cool and serve.

Nutritional Facts Per Serving

- Calories: 62
- Fat: 0g
- Carb: 9g
- Phosphorus: 103mg
- Potassium: 65mg
- Sodium: 62mg
- Protein: 4g

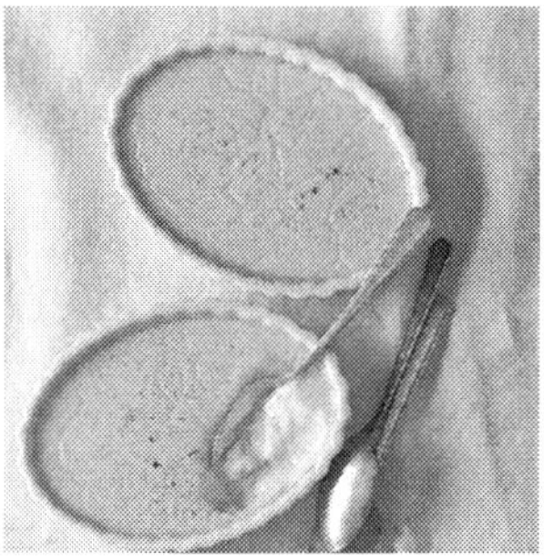

Vanilla Custard

Prep time: 7 minutes	Cook time: 10 minutes	Servings: 10

Ingredients

- Egg – 1
- Vanilla – 1/8 tsp.
- Nutmeg – 1/8 tsp.
- Almond milk – ½ cup
- Stevia - 2 Tbsp.

Method

1. Scald the milk then let it cool slightly.
2. Break the egg into a bowl and beat it with the nutmeg.
3. Add the scalded milk, the vanilla, and the sweetener to taste. Mix well.
4. Place the bowl in a baking pan filled with ½ deep of water.
5. Bake for 30 minutes at 325F.
6. Serve.

Nutritional Facts Per Serving

- Calories: 167.3
- Fat: 9g
- Carb: 11g
- Phosphorus: 205mg
- Potassium: 249mg
- Sodium: 124mg
- Protein: 10g

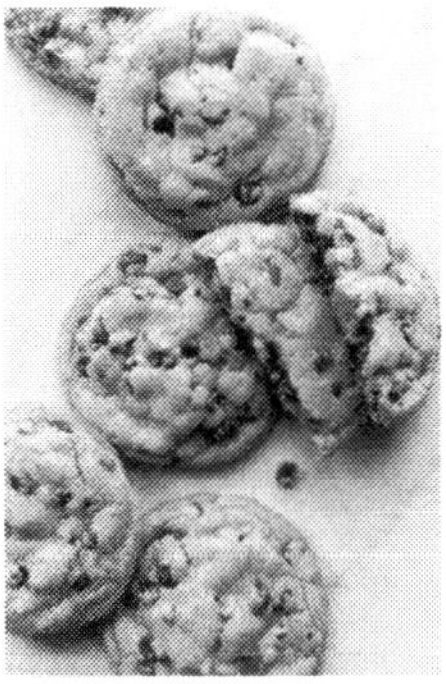

Chocolate Chip Cookies

Prep time: 7 minutes	Cook time: 10 minutes	Servings: 10

Ingredients

- Semi-sweet chocolate chips – ½ cup
- Baking soda – ½ tsp.
- Vanilla – ½ tsp.
- Egg – 1
- Flour – 1 cup
- Margarine – ½ cup
- Stevia – 4 tsp.

Method

1. Sift the dry ingredients.
2. Cream the margarine, stevia, vanilla and egg with a whisk.
3. Add flour mixture and beat well.
4. Stir in the chocolate chips, then drop teaspoonfuls of the mixture over a greased baking sheet.
5. Bake the cookies for about 10 minutes at 375F.

6. Cool and serve.

Nutritional Facts Per Serving

- Calories: 106.2
- Fat: 7g
- Carb: 8.9g
- Phosphorus: 19mg
- Potassium: 28mg
- Sodium: 98mg
- Protein: 1.5g

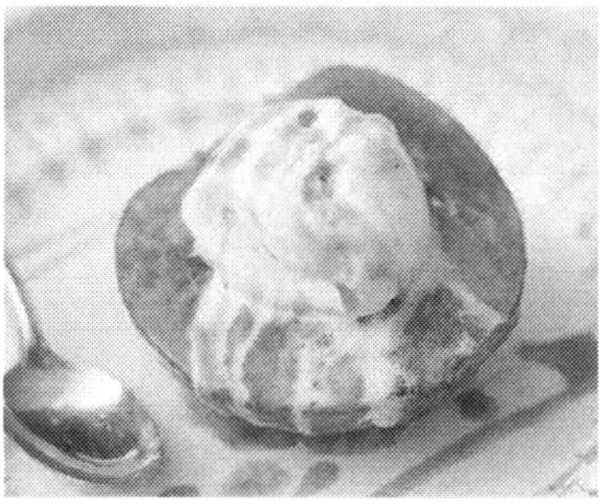

Baked Peaches with Cream Cheese

Prep time: 10 minutes	Cook time: 15 minutes	Servings: 4

Ingredients

- Plain cream cheese – 1 cup
- Crushed meringue cookies – ½ cup
- Ground cinnamon – ¼ tsp.
- Pinch ground nutmeg

- Canned peach halves – 8, in juice
- Honey – 2 Tbsp.

Method

1. Preheat the oven to 350F.
2. Line a baking sheet with parchment paper. Set aside.
3. In a small bowl, stir together the meringue cookies, cream cheese, cinnamon, and nutmeg.
4. Spoon the cream cheese mixture evenly into the cavities in the peach halves.
5. Place the peaches on the baking sheet and bake for 15 minutes or until the fruit is soft and the cheese is melted.
6. Remove the peaches from the baking sheet onto plates.
7. Drizzle with honey and serve.

Nutritional Facts Per Serving

- Calories: 260
- Fat: 20g
- Carb: 19g
- Phosphorus: 74mg
- Potassium: 198mg
- Sodium: 216mg
- Protein: 4g

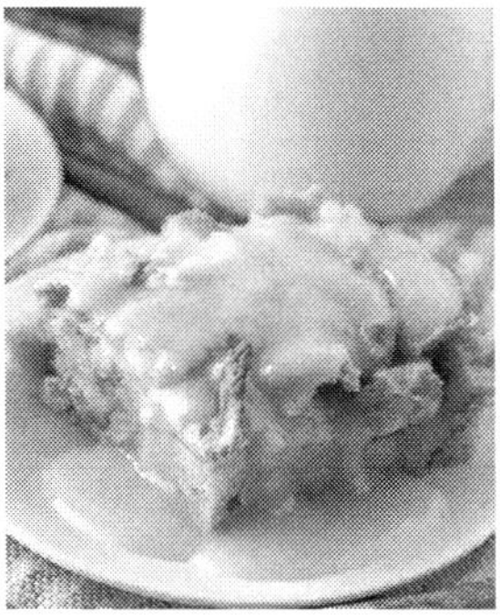

Bread Pudding

Prep time: 15 minutes	Cook time: 40 minutes	Servings: 6

Ingredients

- Unsalted butter, for greasing the baking dish
- Plain rice milk – 1 ½ cups
- Eggs – 2
- Egg whites – 2
- Honey – ¼ cup
- Pure vanilla extract – 1 tsp.
- Cubed white bread – 6 cups

Method

1. Lightly grease an 8-by-8-inch baking dish with butter. Set aside.
2. In a bowl, whisk together the eggs, egg whites, rice milk, honey, and vanilla.
3. Add the bread cubes and stir until the bread is coated.
4. Transfer the mixture to the baking dish and cover with plastic wrap.

5. Store the dish in the refrigerator for at least 3 hours.
6. Preheat the oven to 325F.
7. Remove the plastic wrap from the baking dish and bake the pudding for 35 to 40 minutes, or until golden brown.
8. Serve.

Nutritional Facts Per Serving

- Calories: 167
- Fat: 3g
- Carb: 30g
- Phosphorus: 95mg
- Potassium: 93mg
- Sodium: 189mg
- Protein: 6g

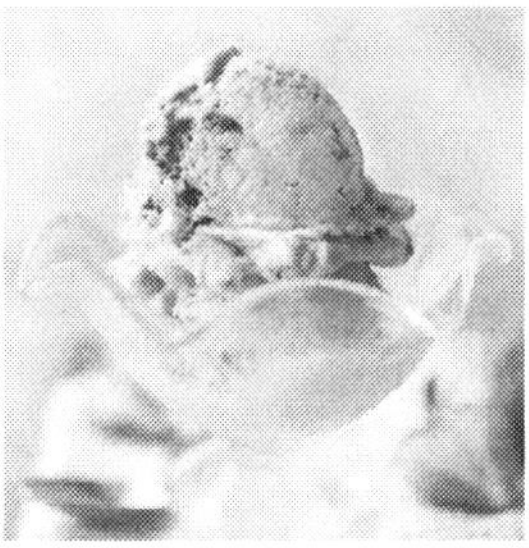

Strawberry Ice Cream

Prep time: 5 minutes	Cook time: 5 minutes	Servings: 3

Ingredients

- Stevia – ½ cup

- Lemon juice – 1 Tbsp.
- Non-dairy coffee creamer – ¾ cup
- Strawberries – 10 oz.
- Crushed ice – 1 cup

Method

1. Blend everything in a blend until smooth.
2. Freeze until frozen.
3. Serve.

Nutritional Facts Per Serving

- Calories: 94.4
- Fat: 6g
- Carb: 8.3g
- Phosphorus: 25mg
- Potassium: 108mg
- Sodium: 25mg
- Protein: 1.3g

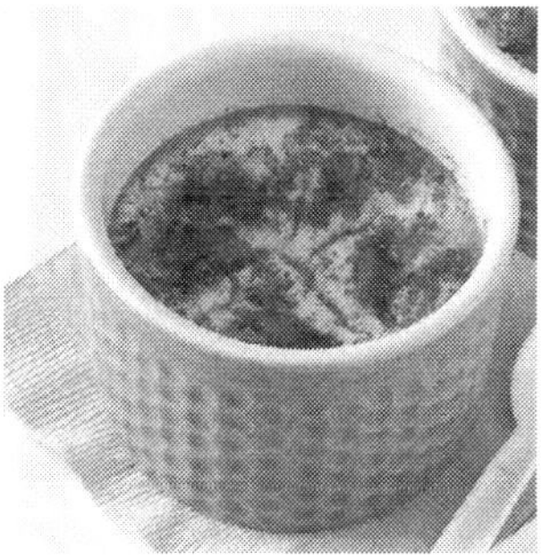

Cinnamon Custard

Prep time: 20 minutes	Cook time: 1 hour	Servings: 6

Ingredients

- Unsalted butter, for greasing the ramekins
- Plain rice milk – 1 ½ cups
- Eggs – 4
- Granulated sugar – ¼ cup
- Pure vanilla extract – 1 tsp.
- Ground cinnamon – ½ tsp.
- Cinnamon sticks for garnish

Method

1. Preheat the oven to 325F.
2. Lightly grease 6 ramekins and place them in a baking dish. Set aside.
3. In a large bowl, whisk together the eggs, rice milk, sugar, vanilla, and cinnamon until the mixture is very smooth.
4. Pour the mixture through a fine sieve into a pitcher.

5. Evenly divide the custard mixture among the ramekins.
6. Fill the baking dish with hot water, until the water reaches halfway up the sides of the ramekins.
7. Bake for 1 hour or until the custards are set and a knife inserted in the center comes out clean.
8. Remove the custards from the oven and take the ramekins out of the water.
9. Cool on the wire racks for 1 hour then chill for 1 hour.
10. Garnish with cinnamon sticks and serve.

Nutritional Facts Per Serving

- Calories: 110
- Fat: 4g
- Carb: 14g
- Phosphorus: 100mg
- Potassium: 64mg
- Sodium: 71mg
- Protein: 4g

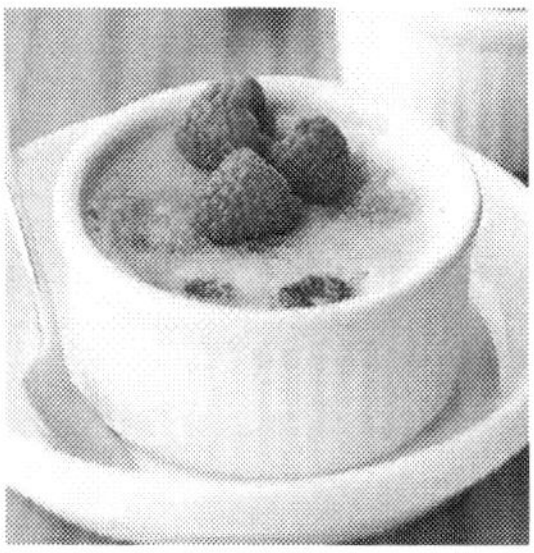

Raspberry Brûlée

Prep time: 15 minutes	Cook time: 1 minutes	Servings: 4

Ingredients

- Light sour cream – ½ cup
- Plain cream cheese – ½ cup
- Brown sugar – ¼ cup, divided
- Ground cinnamon – ¼ tsp.
- Fresh raspberries – 1 cup

Method

1. Preheat the oven to broil.
2. In a bowl, beat together the cream cheese, sour cream, 2 tbsp. brown sugar and cinnamon for 4 minutes or until the mixture is very smooth and fluffy.
3. Evenly divide the raspberries among 4 (4-ounce) ramekins.
4. Spoon the cream cheese mixture over the berries and smooth the tops.
5. Sprinkle ½ tbsp. brown sugar evenly over each ramekin.
6. Place the ramekins on a baking sheet and broil 4 inches from the heating element until the sugar is caramelized and golden brown.
7. Cool and serve.

Nutritional Facts Per Serving

- Calories: 188
- Fat: 13g
- Carb: 16g
- Phosphorus: 60mg

- Potassium: 158mg
- Sodium: 132mg
- Protein: 3g

Conclusion

Adjusting your diet is one of the easiest steps you can take to help alleviate the symptoms of kidncy discasc and avoid dialysis. Being diagnosed with kidney disease can be alarming but you should know that it is still possible to live a healthy life with the help of a renal diet plan. This is more than just an ordinary cookbook. It will give patients a completely new healthy and tasty meal experience. Take your time and enjoy your life without spending much time in the kitchen.

Made in the USA
Columbia, SC
21 December 2022

b2514708-b484-4562-949f-7cd444cb22ccR01